# How to Live with Dying

Tim Zoebelein, M.S.W.

Book Cover by Maureen Zoebelein
Edited by: Ariane Kimlinger at Owl Focus Editing

Print: 979-8-9936450-0-1
eBook: 979-8-9936450-1-8

## Advance Praise for
## *How to Live with Dying*

"*How to Live with Dying* is a beautifully produced volume which provides the deepest depths of experiencing, exploring, and understanding the grief process with fresh insights and profound inspiration and creativity."

-Rabbi Earl A. Grollman, D.H.L., D.D.
Author of *Living When a Loved One Has Died*

"I cannot recall another book like this one in which text and poetry combine to stimulate a reader's thoughts and feelings about the processes that lead up to death and follow after a death. This book is a unique achievement."

-Charles A. Corr. PH.D., Professor Emeritus Southern Illinois University Edwardsville. Author and authority on grief

"*How to Live with Dying* is eloquent and moving ..."

-Dr. Elie Wiesel
Author of *Night* and Nobel Peace Prize Winner

"In a culture which is afraid of dying and death, Tim Zobelein's writing offers reassurance and hope. Because he is comfortable in the presence of those who are dying and those who grieve, he helps us to know that death is a part of life and that life does not end with death. Yet he does not underestimate the pain and anguish of separation and letting go, which is an integral part of death. How to Live with Dying will serve as an instrument of peace and healing."

-Mother Frances Dominica; Speaker, author and founder of Helen House Children's Hospice in Oxford, England

"A simple book with a big message—you can survive a loss! With heartening words, heartfelt poems, and places for your feelings, this book will guide you through your difficult times."

-Allen Klein Author of
*The Courage to Laugh: Humor, Hope and Healing in the Face of Death and Dying*

# Contents

***How to Live with Dying*** is dedicated to the true loves of my life—my wife, Maureen, and my children, Dylan Thomas and Ava Sinead. And in loving memory of my parents, Thomas and Dorothy Zoebelein.

# How to Live with Dying

Tim Zoebelein, M.S.W.

# Introduction

FACING DEATH, WHETHER IT'S your own or that of someone you love, can be like entering a dark room. The purpose of this book is to help guide you through that darkness.

There is a normal progression in death, with a period of time following a death called *bereavement.* As a bereavement counselor and former hospice worker, I've had the opportunity to work with the dying and bereaved for the past thirty-eight years. Even though every situation is different, there are common themes and steps to moving through the course of dying and bereavement. This book attempts to demystify these events by taking you through them a step at a time. I've identified them in four ways:

1. A statement which identifies a task, a state of being, or a question to think about.

2. A discussion of ways to understand and find the tools to deal with dying and bereavement.

3. Poetry—which connects the brain to the heart. To heal, both an intellectual and emotional understanding needs to take place. The poetry is the emotional discussion for each section and is intended to evoke feelings that surround these kinds of experiences.

4. A space to record your own *Observations, Insights, and Remembrances.* If you are dying, think of this as a place to

record some of your thoughts and feelings for yourself or for your loved ones. This can be a place for them to go to for understanding about what you are going through and a place for them to go back to after you're gone. This can become a meaningful family record, part of your family history. Use the written word, drawings, photographs or collage to express your feelings and experiences.

***How to Live with Dying*** was inspired by the individuals and families I've encountered in my work. Most were ordinary people who showed extraordinary courage as they faced their own death or the death of a loved one. I wrote about it as I tried to live with and make sense of all I'd seen.

I began with writing poetry. Each poem in this book reflects my observational journey with those who struggled to cope with death and life. I've tried to strike a balance in this work. It is purposely written with short sections, meant to have enough depth to help the reader develop insights and survive this intense time—without being overwhelmed by a lengthy text.

***How to Live with Dying*** is written for anyone impacted by death:

—Those who are facing their own death
—Those who are accompanying a loved one through the dying process
—Bereaved individuals who are struggling to find their way back into life
—Professionals who deal with dying and bereavement

There are potential insights for all. Insight creates empathy—no matter which role is being addressed in a particular section of the book. The greater the empathy during this unique time in life, the more bearable it will be.

You can read the book in several different ways. You may read it from start to finish. However, dealing with death and healing is often emotionally and physically exhausting—so you may want to read it in pieces. Skip around in whatever fashion is helpful. My sincerest hope is that ***How to Live with Dying*** will serve to comfort and heal.

# Chapter One

## Dying and Death

OUT OF THE MANY mysteries surrounding death, one partially answerable one is how we die. It is the most tangible of the mysteries as it can be seen in what our physical body goes through, and experienced by what we think and feel.

If how we die can be communicated, then what is the mystery? The mystery is that we don't discuss it. This is a time of life that can be talked about. The process of dying is hidden behind a veil of silence, but in sharing our experiences, the veil is lifted.

**This chapter suggests ways through the silence as it discusses the various aspects of dying:**

—Preparing to die.

—Discovering how to be with someone who is ill and will be dying.

—Maintaining a relationship with someone who is sick and at the end of life.

—Responding to the moment of death.

—Knowing what to do for or say to children about the end of life.

—Finding renewed life in the midst of great sorrow.

## Loss Can Leave Us Tongue-tied

### It's sometimes hard to know what to do or say around someone who is dying-even family and friends.

THE PROCESS OF DYING is made up of many losses. Some losses, like physical changes in the body can be anticipated. Others, like newly found emotional distance in close family and friends, are not.

At the end of life, physical and emotional detachment in family and friends nurtures feelings of abandonment. If you find yourself detaching from your loved one, it is important to find ways to stay engaged. You can keep them in your life by teaching yourself how to adjust to the unwelcome presence of the illness in your relationship.

One way to make this adjustment is to rediscover what is still normal. Finding that normal begins by seeing how much or how little things have changed in the way you can relate.

Try reversing roles. What would you need if *you* were the one who was sick and dying? How would you want to be treated? Would you want people near and involved or want them to stay away? What would it be like if lifelong friends became tongue-tied? Would you want to discuss daily events or would you only want to talk about your illness? Would you still value your friendships and savor the moments together? Asking yourself these questions will give you some solid cues for what remains unchanged in how you can interact with your loved one.

Relationships are between people. It is not only important to understand what your loved one's need is for you, it's equally important to understand what your needs are when the two of you are together.

**To develop an awareness of your needs, start by asking yourself these questions:**

—How do I feel to see her so sick?
—What can I do when I think of myself as helpless and inadequate?
—How can I listen to her when I feel uncomfortable and think of her impending death and our separation?
—What can I do when being around her overwhelms me with thoughts of my own death?

Questions like these will help you find a way through your fears by giving you something to truthfully discuss with your loved one. Those fears will become less intense when you have attempted to understand them by answering them together. Unexplored fearful thoughts can overwhelm and immobilize your ability to accept and express love.

The dying of someone close creates an intense time. The intensity can be shaped by thoughts and feelings of abandonment, anger, inadequacy and sadness when your actions are guided by fear. But this time can also be rewarding—filled with openness, hope, friendship, joy and healing when you look to the history of your relationship for guidance—and when your actions are grounded in honest reflection and love.

# SILKEN SCARF

He shuffled like the 96-year-old he is.
From a corner I watched
his hands finger the brim of his hat,
his eyes resting on the shape of his daughter
covered by blankets, dying.
His lips trembled,
his fingertips moved to her soft, fine hair
caressing it as only a father can.
A single tear fell, whispering his love.
She caught it in her silken red scarf, then
with her eyes whispered back,
"I love you, too, Daddy, I love you."

# *Observations, Insights & Remembrances*

# Change and Illness

## Life's routines change with each new progression of an illness.

THINK OF WELLNESS AND illness as if they are on opposite ends of a balancing scale. Initially, the body's health is "heavy" and strong, the illness "light" and in its infancy. Because the scale tips in health's favor, your regular routines in life can be followed as if nothing is wrong. But as the illness progresses, it becomes "heavier" and stronger, reversing direction and tipping the scale in its favor.

Each new progression of the disease has an impact and compromises life's dream in some way. It limits what can be done and makes you ever more dependent. There are medications to take, medical equipment to use, new feelings to deal with, therapies to try and a bevy of professionals to help you. Sometimes all of the changes can be overwhelming.

During those times, find ways to limit your medical activities and increase the things that bring you solace or pleasure. What you have to deal with isn't going away, so it's okay to take a break to rebalance the scale.

**Some ways to do this are:**

—When you are medically able, take a break from healthcare professionals; schedule break days from medical care. Don't be afraid to cancel an appointment and reschedule another day.

—If you can't limit healthcare activities, exercise choice over when your appointments will be. You can group together or separate out different appointments.

How you engage in pleasurable activities also changes with the progression of the illness. As your physical condition changes, you will no longer be able to do the important things you used to. Coming to this realization allows you to begin choosing how you will spend your energy. There's only so much energy in your bank, you can stop doing things that give you little satisfaction. Instead, seek out activities that give you fulfillment and find the ways you are physically able to enjoy them.

**Some changes that can help you adjust to your changing body:**

—Use a wheelchair to go for a walk. You can get the pleasure of the walk without the physical cost of walking.

—Allow others to assist you.

—Use the electric cart at the grocery store or the mall.

—Get a disabled parking permit so you can park closer to essential shopping, the theater, the lake or the fishing hole.

***Don't let the illness prematurely take life away from you.***

## MANDELA

Turning on the TV news,
the rioting has spread to the countryside.
I think of my body and its decay
like a corrupt fifth world dictator
randomly oppressing the enjoyments in life.
In my waking hours,
the fatigue keeps a tireless, ruthless, watch.
My laughter, once easy, bends to its will.
All motion is exhaustion.
I still love, though, in portions.
A slice for my husband. A loaf for my children.
Some crust for me.
These compromises cover me like a scratchy, woolen blanket.
They smother, slowly, all impulses to do
anything or nothing, as I please.
Could I fight, I would, so I yearn for the violence
and the smashing of oppression
the TV news delivers.
Mandela knows my plea.

*Observations, Insights, & Remembrances*

## Remembering Who You Are

Couples often put their needs—to be held, to be intimate— on hold while they struggle with bodies changed by illness, medications, and medical crisis after medical crisis.

Once a couple puts meaningful communication on hold, the distance created by the lack of intimacy becomes difficult to discuss. Intimacy may be awkward, becoming a bother rather than a natural expression of trust and love.

The process of becoming less intimate usually takes place slowly, over time. You may notice yourself feeling increasingly isolated and dissatisfied.

**Signs that intimacy has been put on hold:**

—Keeping things to yourself that you previously would have discussed.

—Seeking the companionship of television, books or movies over that of your loved one.

—Fantasizing about the intimacy you had without making it happen again.

—Shielding your loved one from the very things for which you used to seek him out.

To begin changing this and re-engaging, try remembering how intimate communication and expression happened prior to the illness. How were you aware of your needs for intimacy and how did you address them before the illness forced its way into your relationship?

—Was it when you needed to talk?
—Was it when you wanted to be held?
—Was it when you were thinking or feeling?

If it was through conversation, try talking again. The first step would be trying to talk more often. Increase the time you spend together. When you're ready to withdraw, delay withdrawing. Stay and talk. Even if it's not the same quality of conversation you are used to, it still serves as a connection that emotionally feeds and will be remembered.

If it was by touch, reach out physically in whatever way you can, even if it's only holding hands at the bedside. You can say a lot with just your eyes.

The illness might bring about changes in what you want and what you can do, but it's unlikely it's changed your need to express and receive love.

# YOUR SCENT IS NOT YET A MEMORY

Bald head with flecks of gray,
the chemo burned like napalm.
I caress your skin as if
your soft pony tailed hair still
falls between the triangles of your back.
I reach to push it aside,
for our lovemaking always begins
with caresses and a kiss.

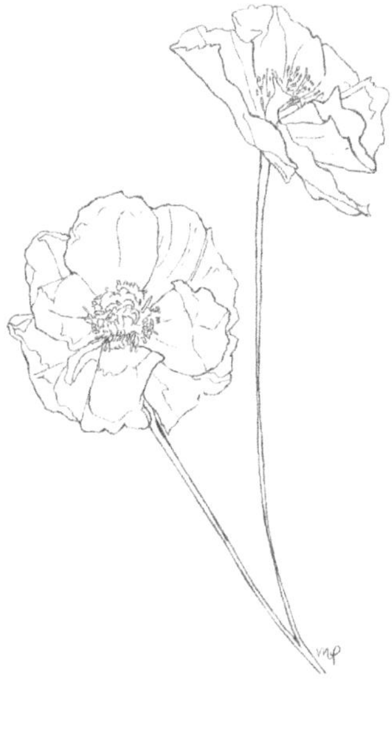

*Observations, Insights & Remembrances*

## Expectations and Learned Anticipations

### What do you think will happen when someone has entered the process of dying?

WHAT GOES ALONG WITH dying and death? We tend to think – *You are sick. Then you die.* The reality is that dying is a process with death being the final event in that process.

We have certain expectations about living. We eat, we drink, and we have the energy to do things. There are normal routines and expectations. A different normalcy develops in the process of dying with different routines to follow. Living with dying, resulting in the changes of everyday activities, will lead you to discover this new "normal."

When you are healthy, normal tasks and pursuits for living a quality life may not be normal for having a quality life when you are ill. Preparing for the changes, and the willingness to develop new expectations, will help you deal with them more effectively.

Dying is like going on a trip down a highway. You don't just arrive at your destination . . . you have to drive there. While driving, your car will get worn and dirty, you'll pass road signs and towns, the road will be smooth in some spots and rough in others.

On your loved one's journey, there will be road signs to indicate when death is near. While they vary with the type of illness, along with the age and sex of the person, there are several universal signs:

—Loss of appetite and a decrease in drinking
—Extreme fatigue
—Withdrawal and mood swings
—Changed interests

Things that were important no longer are. The desire and energy for simple activities goes away as the body winds down from living. It doesn't require food in the same way so appetite decreases until eventually, eating simply stops. Fluid intake decreases. Exhaustion will continually increase.

These changes will occur and they are normal.

If you are caring for a dying person, anticipating these changes allows you to find the new routine and follow it more easily, helping you focus on the things that are really important at the present. If you are the one who is dying, you can more comfortably accept these changes when you know they are coming and are normal at the end of life.

## REMEMBERED FEARS

The chef spread
his corpulent chin
between the fingers of his hands
and cried.
With a youngster's fright
hidden by decades of eating
within his seventy inch waist.
Hidden until this morning,
when staring at his breakfast plate
he found the cancer had dulled his hunger
and taken the desire to eat.

# *Observations, Insights & Remembrances*

## Surrounded by Unrehearsed Change

### What you might anticipate in the final weeks before death might not be what happens.

Often in the natural process of dying, the unexpected can occur. There's no difference in the moment of death. It is what occurs with each body in the time before death that is different. Most hospice programs have a guide that outlines what is common in the course of dying. Although the guide details a wide variety of things that might happen, it is quite typical to screen out those things you can't imagine happening to you or your loved one.

By screening unimaginable things out, you are creating the possibility for a personal crisis.

The key to understanding dying is to know that although much can be predicted, not everything can be. Even those predictable things will still have variations as everyone's body responds to illness in both similar and different ways, making everyone's dying similar, yet different.

**Common events you might not anticipate:**

—Thinking someone is near the end of life, yet surprisingly, he continues to live in a diminished state.

—Thinking you will have time to discuss the things on your mind, but fatigue quickly exhausts him within minutes of starting to talk.

—Expecting bodily functions (e.g. bowel movements) to be kept as private as they've always been, when in reality, they find their way into most conversations— especially dinner conversations.

—Planning to never leave your loved one alone, yet you and she need time apart. She says not to hover/you realize you haven't had time to relax and do what you want.

—Experiencing the unsettling, but potential normal, events leading to the moment of death, which may include:

> —listening to your loved one's loud and gurgling breathing doesn't mean he's struggling.
> —hearing him moan, even when he's comfortable.
> —seeing him stare as if seeing through you.

During the times when the unexpected occurs, allow yourself to redefine what being together means. If lengthy conversations can't happen, quietly sit together and hold hands. If fatigue claims most waking moments, find what can be done when he has energy. When discovering how much you need time away, it's okay to have that time. When bodily functions win out as the topic of conversation, let them. Realize that our primitive human needs become the important ones for comfort when dying.

## YOUNG LOVERS

Death
your death
I never thought would be loud.
I imagined holding your hand
while sitting on a pastel cushioned chair by your bedside.
Communicating love through looks and well-chosen words.
I imagined lifting your head to rest on embroidered pillows that
I'd fluff each hour when I wasn't kissing your brow
or cradling you to sleep.
I imagined, in the final weeks,
saying those things we might have,
had we had a lifetime.
Feeling somehow satisfied
that we'd burned bright, though not long.
I imagined so much in those early days
when we first learned you'd be dying but
never in my darkest thoughts imagined
your death would be loud.
With thundering breaths.
Would be unconscious,
waking, haunted by pain.
Would be cheating the time needed
to sustain our memories.
Would be emptiness coexisting
with sadness and rage
I never thought your death would be loud.

# *Observations, Insights & Remembrances*

## Childhood Isn't Always Peaceful

For many of us, the realization that a child can die is unimaginable and heartbreaking. The discomfort might make us unable to hear our family's needs.

For the friends and caregivers of a dying child and her family, the greatest help you can give is listening and preparing.

Ask what is needed . . . then take time to hear the complete answer. Do what is within your power to do, even if you think it's not what the family needs.

The most significant way you can help a family to prepare is to tell the truth and encourage the family to discuss their concerns openly. If a family or child wants to know something, find a way to tell them, even if you fear that your answer will upset them. Families usually don't ask if they don't want to know.

Respect their needs and choices. Do not decide what a family needs without their input.

If you are a healthcare professional, you can prepare a family by not offering unrealistic hope. Give families information on the best possible care even if that care is no longer curative. Help the child who is sick have a means to express her desires and concerns.

Discussing difficult issues with a family can sometimes be aided by including others in the conversation. You and other family friends can provide support together. Faith community representatives can be a further resource. Healthcare professionals can provide the greatest assistance to the family by utilizing an interdisciplinary team approach; a team that should include social workers, nurses, chaplains and other staff who have bonded with the family.

If you believe you're protecting the family by keeping them from the truth, it's important to remember that these omissions are often based on your need to be protected from your feelings of fear, impotence and sadness. If you discover yourself acting out of your needs and not theirs, find the support you need to help yourself.

## HIS WORK GOES THROUGH ME

In the school hallway
your eyes scanned the floor
not looking, but seeing
the image of your sister, quiet.
The cancer's grip loosened for the first time since
that emergency room Thanksgiving feast of pretzels and Coke
three years ago.
You wanted to be home
not here, waiting for class, knowing she'd died.
When I asked if you'd like to see her,
to be with those you know,
you focused and said, "Yes."
You questioned death
trying to fit it in with living (it wouldn't).
You wanted to be her older sister one last time
before her body was taken.
In your driveway you walked from the car, unsteady,
with the presence of someone grown older.
You sat beside her on the bunk bed and felt her skin.
You ran your fingers over the tumors and through her hair.
Death had spoken.
This is the last talk, the last touch, the last goodbye.
I asked what you'd like to say to her, you said, "I love you."
I asked what you'd like to do and watched you reach
for your favorite doll and tuck it underneath her arm.

We sat, the three of us, until the hearse arrived.
Her six-year-old body barely held down the blanket on which
she was lain.
You melted into me.
My tears ran off my chin and onto your shoulder.

## *Observations, Insights & Remembrances*

## Beliefs About Life Challenged by Death

Weeks to days before death, there are frequently "visits" from loved ones who have already died.

Episodes can occur in the course of dying that are unfamiliar to everyday life and may appear to be mystical and unreal.

In the weeks, days and nights before death, "visits" can occur from loved ones that have died. It can be anyone of importance—a deceased wife or husband, a mother or father, a son or daughter, a friend. The reality of their death is forgotten and they become alive again through a vision or dream.

These visions occur with all kinds of people, in all imaginable situations. They more often occur through dreams when asleep, either during the day or at night, but can sometimes happen when awake as well. Unlike regular dreams that are usually implausible or forgotten, these have the quality of a "visit." They can be remembered in great detail and many times will provide comfort as they reestablish longed-for relationships.

Out of fear, discomfort, or denial, you might want to redirect your loved one's conversation or your own thoughts to some other topic; as if in doing so, you might escape the reality that death is near.

Rather than being afraid when and if your loved one has a "visitation," recognize it and embrace the comfort it can bring. People who mention having such an experience will usually talk about it if you are willing to listen. Discover what this means to you and to your loved one. You can be aware of your feelings that may arise, such as discomfort or disbelief, but try not to trivialize the experience or laugh it off. Rather, accept what your loved one is experiencing, then reflect and talk with others involved—hold hands, listen without judging, and be present.

## SON

Sidewalk and chalk.
The memories are near of the hours
I watched you growing,
of the warmth of your sleep
and breath upon my shoulder.
With smell, and touch, and hearing
the memories live again.
As my lungs heave under the drowning weight of fluid.
As sleep is no longer separated into days by night.
As I get closer to dying
the memories break out to pull at my hand.
Death shines a light on the pathway.
I have only to take the final picture of
the sun-warmed room.
Of the tears on my husband's cheek and
the understanding from 71 years of life.
Of the last kiss.
The sensation of growing cold and
the stiffness of my heartbeat.
I have only to take this final picture before
I break out and run.
Run to you my son. Torn from the living
40 years ago when I was young.
When I was young, the memories that belong to the aged
lived for you. I can finally let them fade.
When I hold you in real time, I can let them fade.
I have only to die for living.

## *Observations, Insights & Remembrances*

# Talking With Children

## How do I talk to my child about death?

Talking with a child about death—whether it be hers or that of someone she loves—can be frightening. It is easy to think there is some missing formula you need to discover. There is no formula. Your relationship with this child and your intuitive understanding of what works in that relationship will give you the guidance you need.

Your job is to help her understand the events happening to her on whatever level she can comprehend. The temptation, when seeing the emotional turmoil of someone who is young, is to think you need to help her flawlessly, to help her perfectly. The problem with perfection is that we're all perfectly imperfect. There is not going to be just one chance to say things correctly.

An ongoing dialogue will probably occur on different levels—both verbal and nonverbal. The ingredients necessary for this communication are honesty, openness and simplicity.

**Elements for ongoing dialogue:**

**Verbal Honesty**

—Tell the truth in every discussion. It doesn't mean you have to give all the intricacies for an adult's level of understanding, but rather, reach out to her with respect for where she is in age and emotional development; pare it down to a level she can handle and understand.

**<u>Nonverbal Honesty</u>**

—Don't mislead in any form. Show your child your own sorrow. It doesn't mean you unload all of your emotional turmoil on her. It *does* mean it's okay to cry. Through your tears, you can let her know that even in sorrow, people can be okay.

**<u>Openness</u>**

—Be alert for opportune moments to talk. Let her know that she can always begin conversations with you.

**<u>Simplicity</u>**

—Continual understanding and patience. Children don't absorb the reality of death in one sitting. She will keep grabbing for small pieces of all there is to comprehend. It might be in one-sentence statements or questions, in a conversation, in the way she plays, in her discussions with friends, in her drawings, or through her actions. These are all ways children process things that are an emotional and intellectual big deal. Don't be misled into thinking that because you initiated a conversation that covered all you wanted to talk about, that it fulfilled her need to integrate and to understand. It probably didn't.

You can't shield her from the pain and sorrow that goes with loss. If you give misleading answers, you'll confuse her. Protecting her in this way might work in the short term, but in the long term it will damage her and undermine your relationship. One day she will know the truth and look back to you for an accounting. Rather than doing the impossible job of shielding her from pain, help her learn what to do with it.

If you become emotionally overwhelmed and unavailable, appoint someone she can go to whom you both love and trust. Let her know that sometimes you might not be able or ready to talk. At those times, she needs to know she is safe by having someone else to talk with. Together, you will need to decide who that person is going to be.

You're not always going to get it right. Through love and trust, you will get a second, third and fourth chance.

## AM I DOING SOMETHING WRONG?

He told the lie to his children
that the ocean winds
on days of gray storm clouds
were there to carry their tears
on billowing rain
to the sorrowless
Land of Forgetting.
They grew up believing.
Always tested
by the ever-present pain
born from his lie,
nurtured in silence,
that gnawed inside.

## *Observations, Insights & Remembrances*

## Fearing Loss of Control and Choice

### I've heard people say they're not afraid of death, they're afraid of dying.

Perhaps you are faced with the fear that your illness is going to leave you without choices and feeling out of control. You might have drawn the conclusion that ending your life is the only answer, the only way to retain your control and dignity. This is not an uncommon thought.

But there is another choice, known as hospice. Good hospice care gives you and your family the resources and skills to gain control over the symptoms of your illness. Hospice aggressively focuses on comfort during the dying process, along with providing emotional and spiritual support for you and those you love.

Choices on how to control symptoms and receive support are presented to you. You choose what you do and do not want. As your needs for comfort evolve in response to the changes of the illness, the level of support provided by hospice can change to meet your needs; hospice strives to respect your understanding of what is right for you. Its goal is to allow you to have what control you can as you wrestle with the end of life.

With hospice care, you can be assured that your pain will be effectively and compassionately managed, and that you, your family and friends will be offered ongoing support. When the symptoms of your illness are managed and you have the support you need, it's possible to have some control during the process that leads to death.

Through comfort care and love, this can be a profound time—a time that affirms relationships, and helps you and those you love prepare for your death.

# 57 YEARS A LONER

Before
I lose my mind,
give me
the clarity
to end my life.
My reliance
on you
is too great.
To wipe myself
is an Olympic event
Was I ever a sports fan?
NO!

## *Observations, Insights & Remembrances*

## Listening to Yourself

### I feel afraid when I imagine the moment of her death.

Even in the best circumstances, fear of the unknown can be a mixture of anxiety and exhilaration. Fear associated with death can be overwhelming—whether it's your own death or the death of someone you love. A key to understanding your fears and expectations of the moment of death is to pay attention to the images that fill your mind.

**Close your eyes and think about these images that might be influenced by several factors:**

—Stories you've heard from others
—Spiritual beliefs
—Television programs or movies
—Your past experiences with death
—Books

But death doesn't always occur in a predictable way. It isn't always going to be how you've seen it in the media, or even personally witnessed before. These are only some of the ways your expectations might have taken root.

Take some time for yourself to discover what you anticipate.

Now, think about the possibilities. There are an infinite number of possibilities, but only a limited number of probabilities. Because you can imagine possible ways death might occur doesn't make what you imagine more probable. What is probable can be found by ruling out the unlikely from your list of possibilities. If you get stuck, bring your list into the next doctor's appointment and discuss it with them. Get a list of signs and symptoms from your local hospice program and compare your list with theirs. Seek out others who have gone through this to talk about your questions and fears. If you focus on what is probable, this time will be more manageable.

## PRAYER

You were dying.
What should I say for the last words you would hear?
I said, "Everything is okay"
and held your hand.
"Everything is okay,
you're a good person."
You relaxed.
The process of dying ended.
I said, "Safe passage."
Still holding your hand
I heard my voice
remembering forgotten prayers from when I was young,
still holding your hand,
I prayed them aloud to you.

*Observations, Insights & Remembrances*

# The Intensity of a Child's Death

## When I think of this child dying, I know I will break. How can I learn to live, to let go?

THE DEATH OF A child, whether she's five days old or twenty-five years old, is like no other loss. It is tender, gentle and so overwhelmingly sad. It's like the abyss that all the combined tears from all of life's losses fall into. It splits the heart from how life should be into the unimaginable reality of how tragic life can be.

To be present with a family and a child at death, though, can be a gift like no other. It's a gift of intimacy to experience this very private moment with them because raw grief strips away social convention and pretense. It leaves the human heart standing naked before all of you.

Witnessing the occurrence of the unfathomable in life, like the death of a child, heightens an awareness of life's sinews. What has been grouped together and taken for granted separates into the awareness of how unique the qualities of our lives are.

Our health and the health of our loved ones become treasured and measured for the time left. The quality of the relationships with our loved ones becomes even more important. The lives of our children are not as easy to take for granted. The adage that a child outlives his parent has been shown to be circumstantial and unreliable as a hard and fast rule.

Being with a family during the death of a child means first looking to the family's needs, then to your own. Be attentive to what they want and need to do to process this time. Family members often need to hold their child—sometimes for hours. If the child is a baby or toddler, his diaper might be changed; his best outfit put on.

Families might still need to talk to him and cry over him. There might be a need to tuck him in, or surround him with favorite toys; to cut a lock of hair or a fingernail to save.

Some family members might need to stand away; to take some time to relive how the death occurred, perhaps even re-enact the child's final words, sounds, and breaths. Others may want to pray with a group in another room, or start making phone calls.

It is important to pay attention to the family's needs without acting out of your own inner agenda. You may want to help, but feel overwhelmingly inadequate. When there is a situation that has great sorrow and need, we often want to help and "do something." But doing something may be standing silently to the side, being ready to help when you see the need.

Stay with your child, no matter her age. Be with her as long as you need to. Just because her body doesn't possess life anymore, doesn't mean you are ready to let go. Hold her, rock her, comb her hair, wash her; do what your instincts tell you.

Don't let her body go until you are ready. When her body is gone, only memories will remain. It's okay to stay with her as long as you need to. After all, she was yours as much as she was her own.

## DAVID

She held him
to the soft time of her breast
and let her heart
beat for his
tasting his scent
in the folds of her skin.
His fingers touched
her sorrow
that entered like a wind
fresh from the darkness
of a starlit wheatfield
or a burdened soul.
He didn't cry
but she did
knowing he was lost to the comfort
she longed to give
though longing cut dully
she couldn't stop
feeling the injustice each time.
She was his mother
and he the dream
that knew he was dying
at one year old or six months or five.
He was old and she was learning
his lessons for caring
on ordinary days
when life thinks it still has tomorrow
and the mundane glows
like a cut glass jewel.

Waiting for emeralds
gives you nothing for all.
Of this she would need to remember
for future times when her hunger needed him near.
So she cradled him lovingly
and bathed him with tears
tasting his scent in the folds of her skin
for a far off day
when her hunger needed him near.

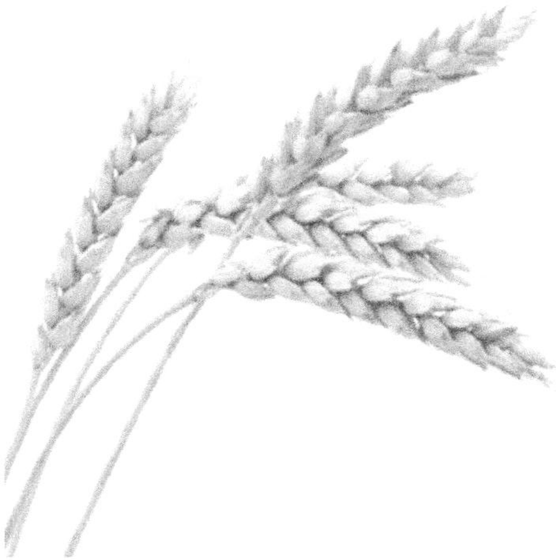

# *Observations, Insights & Remembrances*

# Dying Makes Us All Equal

## Finding the value in your relationships.

It is possible to amass monetary wealth in life, yet no matter how much one has, money doesn't have the power to buy away death. The true value of what we have accumulated in life will manifest itself when entering the final months, weeks and days of life. It's at this time that we each must struggle with what our living and dying means—regardless of our status in life. We will cope with this time leading to death just as we have coped with life. Monetary wealth will fade in importance as you review the value of life's relationships for affirmation or regret.

It isn't too late to invest in changing your relationships—no matter how near or far you are from dying. If you are close, the ways you reach out to people makes a difference. Your gestures and words to include and show kindness will impact those around you and help erase the hardships that are ever-present.

**Some ways to do this are:**

—Showing your appreciation and saying thank you

—Asking about the well-being of those who are important to you

—Trying to help in whatever ways you can—which may simply involve allowing others to help you

—Listening

Even if your relationships have been strained, healing can take place.

If you are not close to dying, you can commit anew to bringing more substance to life's relationships. This will contribute to a happier life and a more peace-filled death when the time draws near.

## KATHY

When my cousin died
I couldn't sleep
so I dreamt of stories
filled with her short shining brown hair
and freckled face squinting in the darkness
of everyday life and seeing, I think.
Stories narrated with her laughter
and easy ways that were so grown-up
even though she was seven years younger she knew.
Stories of her in a party dress
with grass stained knees from chasing the dog
and falling with the rest of us into dandelion dreams.
Stories of her adult life
I hardly knew as a mother and friend
and wife who tried to bring the cancer
to another path that didn't lead to her
and loved despite the fear of it all.
Stories that kept true the understanding
of how we're still kids
costumed with the fabric of age, but inside
giddy and laughing.
When my cousin died
I couldn't sleep
so I dreamt the stories of living
and knew that life was one step closer
to being a dream, a time on the hump of a camel.
When my cousin died
I couldn't sleep, but I knew.

# *Observations, Insights & Remembrances*

## Looking Back on Life and Making Peace

### How do I prepare to die?

If you are terminally ill, preparing to die involves looking inside to your emotional and thinking self, looking out to those you love, and actualizing your faith and spirituality. If the thoughts and actions involved in preparing to die become too emotionally overwhelming, then your body and the growing impact of the illness on your body will prepare you.

Preparing to die involves identifying what you have accomplished in life, and understanding what you still need to do. Taking steps, even little steps, will bring you closer to peace, while taking no steps may keep you stranded in turmoil.

Look inside yourself. You'll want to see and measure what you have accomplished in life.

**Questions to ask yourself:**

—Do you have lingering or unfinished dreams?

—What do you need to say to or do with people who are important to you?

—What things do you want to give to or create for people you love?

After reflecting on these questions, you may want to communicate with the people you care about. Take what has been an internal discussion, and make it external by talking or writing.

Preparing to die is always emotional, and it may be overwhelming.

**Some of the thoughts you may be having if you are emotionally overwhelmed:**

—I'm afraid to die.
—I'm not ready to die now.
—I'm really not terminally ill—I'm just sick.
—A cure will be discovered for what I have, so let's not talk about it anymore.

When you are emotionally overwhelmed and not able to do the work involved in preparing to die, then your body will prepare you. (It will become tired and its weariness will prepare you to concede to death.) From its tiredness will come your readiness to give in to dying.

Regardless of what you have or haven't done, your body will let you know when it is time. In most instances, it will bring you an ever-increasing peace from your emotional and physical struggle. The body's main tools are exhaustion and fatigue. As your illness progresses, they will keep claiming more of you and your time. What you might be able to do today, you won't be able to do tomorrow, or next week, or next month.

The struggle "to do" is then transformed into a desire only "to be."

Finally, even to be alive becomes too much. Soon after, death–no longer the enemy–becomes a welcome friend.

If you are watching someone go through this, the exhaustion that accompanies dying can be unsettling. If you grow impatient or afraid as you see your loved one withdrawing and doing less, understand that the impact of the illness on their body is causing this.

As your loved one gets closer to dying, there will be increasing times when he doesn't appear to be present. The illness causes him to withdraw from you in steps. There will be fewer and shorter times that he will talk. When he looks at you, it might feel like he sees right through you. If this happens, be sensitive to your own emotional needs and reach out to him in whatever ways you can.

Pretend it is six months after his death. Is there anything you would have wanted to do or tell him? If there is, then do it now, while there is still time.

**Identify any spiritual work you'll want to do, which can involve many potential activities:**

—Personal prayer, or praying with others
—Meditation in quiet places or nature
—Visiting your church, temple, mosque, or any other place that holds meaning for you

Spiritual preparation doesn't just happen—it involves your active efforts in reaching inside to your beliefs, then bringing them outside to your living. This is the actualization of your faith.

**Questions to help guide you:**

—How can my spiritual beliefs help me identify ways to help myself, my loved one, others?
—How can my spiritual beliefs prepare me for the death of my loved one?
—What do I believe about death?
—If I need to, whom can I talk to about my spiritual concerns regarding death?

## SILENT

Jo dreams of how she ran
along the paths of the forest park.
Her skin and muscles
had memory then.
Her eyes
were open to the changing sky.
Jo remembers
as the two helpers turn her north,
the direction of her independent, other life,
a four-mile run to the park.
Her weight from lying for months
has brought open wounds
to the skin that held her runner's muscles.
It gathers beside protruding bones
like the moss beside the rocky paths
of the forest park
she dreams.

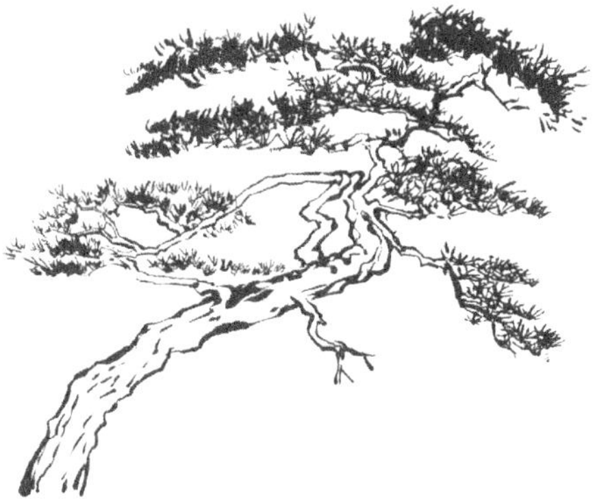

## *Observations, Insights & Remembrances*

## Observations on End of Life

### What happens at the moment of death?

You know your loved one as a living person. The first actual experience of his not living might seem unreal, where the first emotional experience of his death is both emotionally and physically shattering. It is also the beginning of your changed life and your search for a new "normal." You won't know how your future is unfolding, but it is.

The way the moment of death occurs has an endless number of scenarios. Your preparation for this moment depends on the circumstances of the death—whether it comes at the end of an illness, or if it's sudden or tragic. If death is after a long illness, then you probably have been mentally rehearsing for it.

The remarkable quality in the majority of deaths resulting from an illness, is how natural dying is. Unlike what we see in the media and the drama that goes with it, dying comes at the end of a process. The process varies in how breathing changes and how alertness fades into a coma or coma-like state. The normal activities of living, such as eating and drinking, are no longer a necessity. It's as if the body is closing shop, turning out its lights, one by one, at the end of its day.

Although this can sound scary, it usually isn't. It just happens. You can see and hear it happening. Breathing changes, then stops. Life stops. There is silence. You will know it when it happens. Even after the last breath, stay with your loved one for as long as you need to.

## TIME OF DEATH

Two breaths, then, silence,
your heart beat against the aged skin of your neck.
One breath more, no breaths, silence,
your heart continued to beat
an eighty-year habit of guarding life's door.
It seemed to say, in disbelief, "Must it end?"
before it beat no more.

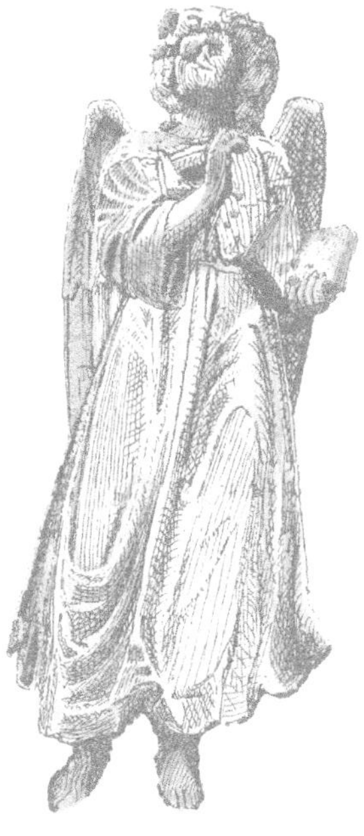

*Observations, Insights & Remembrances*

# Sudden Loss

## How can I cope if my loved one's death is sudden or tragic?

If death occurs suddenly or tragically, you can't prepare for the death, you can only deal with its aftermath. It's like waking to an unwanted dream, only to discover time and again that the dream is real.

To deal with this type of loss, begin by asking how. Gather all of the information you can about the event that claimed his life. After finding out how he died, you may need to spend time with his body; it doesn't matter what condition it's in, he is still the person you love.

Spending time with his body can help you make the emotional connection that death has occurred. It is okay to touch or hold him. Do whatever you need to do for as long as you need to do it. In most instances, you will know when you are ready to move to the next step by letting his physical body go.

If there is no body remaining, you are faced with one of the most difficult losses. Sometimes people disappear through murder, catastrophic accidents and tragedies like Hurricane Katrina or the 9/11 attacks.

When beginning to deal with losses like these, retaining hope that he has somehow managed to survive, or that his body will be found, is important. Hope can be a bridge from the relationship that was, to your relationship with the memories and spirit that remain.

**Begin to regain a sense of control over this unmanageable time in life by taking actions that allow you to grieve:**

—Go as close to the site of death as you can–he was there for his last moments so you can try to find a connection. You might consider taking something from the site to hold onto like a rock, a vial of seawater, or a piece of concrete. You may choose to place your memento in a safe spot, carry it around with you, or incorporate it into your own memorial. You could transform it into art to be worn or displayed. The symbolic action of connecting with your loved one in the last place he lived can be powerful and healing.

—Have a ceremony for closure. Listen to yourself for what creates closure for you. If others are involved, ask them to do the same and discuss your ideas. If you have a funeral with a casket, items can be placed inside it that symbolize your loved one for you: a special or everyday piece of clothing he wore; things he used or touched; objects that symbolize your collective faith; or maybe letters, notes or pictures. When the casket is closed for burial or cremation, the remembrances you've put inside will recreate his essence and offer snapshots to remember his presence in your life.

You and those you love might bring together favorite pictures and organize them into a display. The display can include any items that are important to you for recreating the kind of person he was. You can invite friends and family to view the display with you. This gathering can be a party to celebrate his life or a memorial to commemorate it. It can take place anywhere that holds meaning for you and your loved one; whether it be a place of worship, a restaurant, a favorite park or outdoor spot, or at home.

Discovering how the death occurred, and the ceremonies you develop to remember his life, will enable you to connect with your loss. By allowing yourself to connect with your loss and grieve, paradoxically, your sorrow will become an ever-distant companion.

## LOST

Did you see
the bodies falling?
Did you know it would be you?
Did you feel pain, cry out,
pray, call my name? Did you feel pain?
I do—remembering the times that could have been more
like those of lovers newly discovered
I do—thinking too much or
too little waiting for you to re-appear.
I anticipate loneliness and curl up,
staring out but seeing inside, asking
did you feel pain or call my name
or remember our life as yours was fading?
Could I have done anything that would have kept you
an extra moment but didn't?
Could I, did you, how can, will I,
did you, did you, did you feel pain or suffer?
I know I am
in pale comparison.
I know I've a lifetime for recreating what wasn't broken.
Rebuilding on the blistered wasteland of my deepest heart.
First, I must know,
did you feel pain or cry out my name?
How much of an undertow was your despair when nothing
changed?

## *Observations, Insights & Remembrances*

# Chapter Two

## Search for Meaning

THERE CAN BE A great void in the aftermath of a loved one's death, where initially, little makes sense; so emptiness, confusion and darkness often accompany this loss.

Without sense or purpose, there can appear to be no way out. This chapter helps identify and guide you through the questions that need to be asked during this time of sorrow.

**These questions deal with:**

—Understanding your grief.

—Understanding some of the needs of children at events like funerals.

—Identifying your expectations—then dealing with your true needs during the holidays.

With the right questions, you can create structure to understand your feelings of emptiness. With understanding, you discover the beginning of the way out. This is still a difficult time, but there is hope.

## Different Ways to Grieve

### Is it okay if I grieve differently from you?

**Grieving involves several realizations:**

—Realizing the person you loved has died
—Understanding your struggle to live without him
—Remembering your life has a future

The grief work one person does to gain these realizations can look different from the work of another. Grief work means you're able to identify what you need when you're dealing with the emotional intensity that loss brings. You may need to cry, sleep, talk, write, create, travel, or be with family. It can be almost any internal or external reaching—from feeling, to reflecting, to doing. Not only do you need to identify your needs, but you must also trust yourself; follow your instincts for where your grief work needs to begin.

Within a single family or a close-knit group, there will be differences in grieving based on how each member responds to emotional issues. The two major ways of grief response are feelings—called *intuitive grieving*; and thinking—called *instrumental grieving*.*

## INTUITIVE GRIEVING

Intuitive grieving involves strong feelings that make it difficult to think. Thinking takes a backseat as the emotional turmoil is felt.

Although it might seem the opposite is true, the most important way of processing these feelings is by facing them. Learn their names and come to understand their messages. By sorting through your feelings, you can begin to reclaim yourself.

**Ways to confront emotions as an intuitive griever:**

—Talking and crying with family and friends.
—Joining a grief group.
—Exercising.
—An act of physical aggression, e.g., safely smashing unneeded objects, or beating pillows (*REMEMBER, IT'S NOT OKAY TO HURT YOURSELF, OTHERS, OR ANY LIVING CREATURE*).
—Screaming (in an understanding space).

Remember the goal is to hear and understand. By giving your sorrow an avenue for expression, you're allowing yourself to heal and live again.

With this intuitive style of grieving, people have to make sense of the feelings inside of them to make sense of the world outside.

## INSTRUMENTAL GRIEVING

Unlike the dynamics of intuitive grieving, the instrumental griever processes their loss primarily by thinking and doing. Walking the path of thoughts and tangible actions will bring them closer to a new and changed life.

**Here are some helpful actions an instrumental griever might take:**

—Organizing a remembrance, be it a funeral or gathering.
—Building something for the funeral, like a casket.
—Starting a foundation in memory of who has died.
—Starting a nonprofit.
—Organizing yearly events to raise money for nonprofits.
—Writing a book on their experience (like this one) with loss.

For these grievers, instrumental actions allow them to reach their loss and give it meaning; they need to create actions outside of themselves in order to make sense of their feelings inside.

It's sometimes still believed that if a person doesn't cry as part of their dealing with a loss, then they are in denial. But in reality, not crying is likely following the inborn process that goes with instrumental grieving. In terms of feelings, let's imagine the two processes as color: Intuitive feelings are composed of intense, vibrant colors, much like I think of in Central American folk art. Whereas instrumental feelings would consist of softer pastel shades, quieter and more subtle. The feelings are definitely there in the background, but most of their energy is processed by thinking and doing.

Knowing which of these two ways you tend to process emotions can help you understand the dominant way in which you'll grieve. If you're an intuitive griever, listen to your feelings to make sense of the world; you'll probably need to cry often, talk, hug, reflect, feel with great intensity and revisit those feelings again and again. If you think and act as a way to grasp what you need and understand what you feel, or, instrumentally grieve, you'll probably be the one to call the relatives, organize the funeral and decide on the program. You might work, read, and think. When you resolve one grief issue, you'll not routinely go back to it; you'll go on to the next.

As you might guess, the fundamental differences between these two grief processes have the potential to create conflict, which can be particularly heightened when both styles exist within the same family.

**The person who mainly copes by *feeling* might question why the *thinking* person isn't impacted emotionally:**

—Why is he hiding his emotions?
—Why did he cry a lot at first and now does so infrequently?
—Why doesn't he want to keep going back and reliving the death?
—Why does he talk about this death so logically and constantly want to do things?
—Why does he keep reading and looking for a formula for grief?

Essentially, the person who processes grief primarily by *feeling* wonders why the grieving person who copes mostly by *thinking* is so different.

**And the person who grieves more by *thinking* might not understand why the person who processes more through *feeling* seems stuck, and develops concerns of her process:**

—Will she become lost in her grief?
—Why didn't she experience the same kind of closure he did after the memorial service?
—Why does she keep bringing up the same events when they're over and have already been dealt with?
—Why doesn't she gain the same help he did by reading a particular book?

The person who processes by *thinking* thinks grief should go in a straight line. When you're finished with a piece of grief work, move on! The person who processes by *feeling* understands the interconnection of many lines that have all been altered by the death, and therefore are naturally included, again and again from different angles, in the work of grief.

Many people are neither solely a thought processor or a feeling processor; but are a combination of the two. Think of a continuum—on one extreme end is the *thinking griever*; on the other end, the *feeling griever*. You might find you possess traits from both ends. One might be more dominant than the other, without being exclusive.

**Look at the lists below and circle the traits that fit you:**

## Instrumental

- Thinking
- Feel less intensely
- Guided by thinking things out
- Look for solutions
- Prefer grief class over grief group
- Would like a book with solutions
- Journaling thoughts and some feelings
- Desire to do and work

## Intuitive

- Feeling
- Feel intensely
- Guided by feelings
- Feelings first, solutions later
- Prefer grief group over grief class
- Would like to cry and talk
- Journaling feelings and some thoughts
- Re-engaging in work and doing things occurs over time

If you are almost exclusively on one end of the grief continuum or the other, you have discovered that you're either instrumental or intuitive. If you have circled items from both sides, you are a *blended griever*. Your grief style and subsequent grief work need to encompass tasks from both grieving styles.

Instinctively, if each of you remains unaware of your own and other family members' grief process, you might think your loved one is emotionally scary, lacking, and sometimes even suffering from denial. This will lead one grief style to neutralize the other. When the *feeling* processor becomes emotional, the *thinking* processor seeks to calm her by becoming more logical. When the *thinking* processor doesn't show his emotions, the *feeling* processor tries to "open him up" by expressing her emotions even more. Rather than accomplish the desired effect of bringing your loved one out of denial and closer to your style, neutralizing actions will instead push each other into greater isolation, the outcome being the opposite of what is instinctually needed.

When you can identify your style in emotional work and grieving, you can better tune into your grief needs. When you can appreciate the other person's style, especially when it's different, you no longer need to rescue—you can respect. *Remember that neither style is better*. The most important grief task is to tune into how you need to take care of yourself and take the risks to do what you need to, even when it's different from those around you.

* To further investigate these concepts, go to the book, *Men Don't Cry, Women Do: Transcending Gender Stereotypes of Grief*, by Terry L. Martin and Kenneth J. Doka

## SUNG LOW

I thought it wasn't true
the hoop was too high and you mostly jumped low
I thought you sent me news
about the sullen earth
when we weren't warm
for laughter.
I thought if I smiled
I'd find a way back to any path
that might lead me.
I didn't care about the music so
didn't hear
they were funeral songs.
I thought, not you, ever!
Your love was too robust
too knowing
and patient even when
I failed to embrace
what we both knew was sacred.
I thought you'd last and
I'd be gone.
I should have heard they were funeral songs
sung low.

## *Observations, Insights & Remembrances*

## Seemingly Unending Grief

### How will I ever get through this grief?

**Begin by asking yourself questions about your life and your handling of loss:**

—What was my relationship with the person who died? (Parent, spouse, child, friend, relative or acquaintance)
—What did the relationship mean to me? Did I love, like, dislike, hate, or possibly even fear this person?
—Is my security endangered with this death? Will I lose my house? Will I now struggle financially?
—How did the family I grew up in handle loss and death? Was death talked about? What expectations did my family have for me when someone died?
—Is it okay to feel? With the possible intensity of what I'm feeling, can I carry my responsibilities and make it through the day, week or month?
—Do I have people available who care about me and will I talk with them?

These questions are a starting point for understanding how you might be impacted by your loss. If it's too hard to ask and answer them, look for professional support. You can join a bereavement support group or obtain professional counseling. Wanting to heal is good. Don't be afraid to seek out and use assistance in your healing.

The death of someone loved, and the healing process that follows, is similar to breaking a leg. At first you might not be able to walk; you'll be in shock and feel numb. But, just as your leg progresses with healing, so will you find yourself increasingly able to manage your life, as you learn to live with your loss and work on healing. Eventually, although the break will always be a part of you, you can regain the active use of your leg. Similarly, your sorrow will be a memory you'll encounter rather than a daily reality you live.

# THE FUTURE WHISPERS

Sadness knows a grieving heart,
what was dreamed will be not.
The weekend picnics at a lake-shored park,
firefly catching in glass bottles at dark.
The infant cradled in knowing arms,
the forever task of keeping her from harm.
Dancing to music in stocking feet,
from loving the knowledge of what is complete.
Death is a waking from the dreams to be,
gone is tomorrow for the heart that grieves.

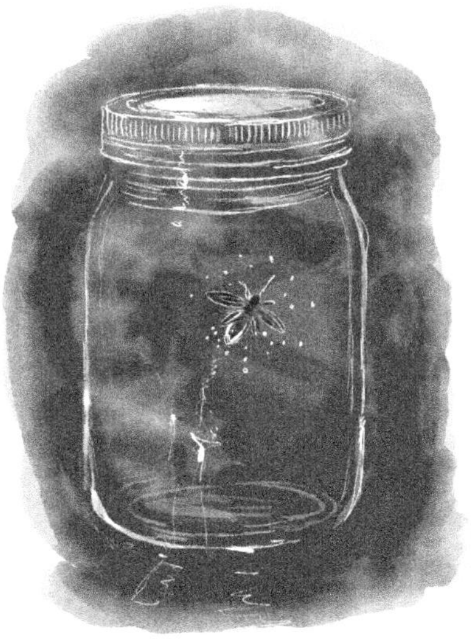

## *Observations, Insights & Remembrances*

## Helping Children

### How can I prepare my children for "what happens" when someone dies and understand what their needs might be after the death of someone known and loved?

You will be your child's first teacher about death. It is possible to help him find meaning within the devastation by guiding him. Through meaning, comes healing.

The first step involves including your child in planning an organized remembrance of your loved one, such as a funeral or memorial gathering. Remembrances like these are vital for integrating loss.

Think of this event as a different version of other family events. Just as you wouldn't exclude or try to protect your child from family gatherings like Thanksgiving, you don't need to exclude or protect him from the memorial gathering. The key is not to protect, but to prepare and include.

**There are several ways to do this:**

—Give him the opportunity to have a role in the planning of the event. The role should be in keeping with his age and ability. He could pick an article of clothing for the deceased to wear or place a special remembrance in the casket. He might choose some of the photographs to display in a memorial gathering. Or, he might help to decide on a kind of memorial plaque or bench, including its location for placement. He could select, a piece of music for the memorial gathering or sing a song.

—Prepare him, based on his age and emotional awareness, for what he might see at the viewing or funeral. Include a description of what will happen and what he might see adults doing when they express grief. This preparation allows him to ask any questions he needs to. Don't be surprised if the same questions are asked over again.

—Let him know that whatever he feels capable of doing is okay. If he needs to leave early, that's fine. If he needs to get close to the casket and touch the body; or in the case of a cremation, wants to handle the urn or touch the ashes; it's okay. If he wants to maintain distance, that's alright too. There is a healthy, natural curiosity about death that can lead children to ask questions and take actions that adults are too restrained to ask about or do.

—Have an emotionally available adult present for your child. This individual can be a family member or friend, and needs to be someone you and he trust; to whom he can go to if his parents are unavailable physically or emotionally.

Involve your child, be open to his questions and needs, and prepare him for the events that will take place. Above all, love him.

## GRAMPS

Your 82 years stretched backward
to water holes and horse drawn carts.
To the nineteenth century
when my father was not.
I was born before your 70th year.
My life securing a place for yours in the future.
I grew up listening as you pecked on a Morse code key.
Explained the glow of a vacuum tube,
and our heritage in the German nobility.
You showed me how to saltwater fish.
To check pay phones for forgotten dimes,
and find flat rocks to skip across the bay.
We'd watch them slip
through the watery veil into shared memory.
Holding your hand, I watched and listened but remained
unaware that you'd grown frail.
The hair on your arms longer
than the width of bone and skin that held them.
On your 82nd birthday, when I was 14,
I searched Main Street's stores for a present
that matched the glow in your eyes and found
a polka dot tie that could shame all colors into trying harder.
Proving true love, you wore it proudly.
Floating on the skies of your drab brown sweater and shirt.
A rainbow ending near the blue treasure of your eyes.
Some short weeks later on the day you died,
in my thinking sorrow when tears stayed back for a little while,
I remembered the polka dot tie
and how you said it looked so sharp.

I realized it had been and so should be my final offering.
Looking at your body dressed in your elegant best clothes.
The polka dot tie draped around your neck stating clearly
that we were friends. I watched as people came near,
and seeing the tie, smiled through their sorrow.
I looked to see it floating, ending
near the blue treasure of your eyes.
But your eyes and life were closed and silent, so
I closed my eyes and remembered.
In remembering, I cradled your life
as it lived on within me.
Securing its place in the future.

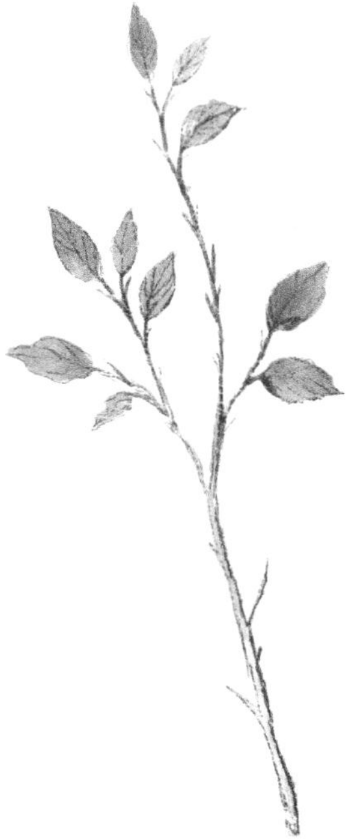

## *Observations, Insights & Remembrances*

## Sudden and Unexpected Death

In many deaths, but especially in sudden, unexpected deaths, there are the questions of why, if and how.

**THE QUESTIONS OF *WHY*, *if*, and *how*, wear many hats:**

—*Why didn't he ...?*
—*If only I ...*
—*How come she ...?*

It's important to ask these difficult questions and appreciate what asking them might mean.

Asking these questions serves the hidden purpose of helping keep in place what used to be. Each time you ask, you create the momentary hope you can discover a way to alter the events that caused his death. Momentary hope is like a salve that numbs the full pain of your loss by emotionally giving you time to adjust to his physical absence from your life.

The time will come when it's important to take the next step toward realization. The realization that for whatever reason, he or she has died. Strong feelings—emptiness, loneliness, sadness—can often accompany this realization. Even though you cannot go back and redo whatever happened that caused the death, you can deal with your feelings. It's not easy, but necessary for the healing process.

Instead of persisting in trying to undo your loss, think of facing what it is and what it means to you. Try experimenting with how you can accommodate yourself to the challenges of living your changed life; one forever altered by this loss. It can still be filled with promise through the intertwining of past, present, and future.

## PARENTS' NIGHTMARE

My son drowned last year
while I sat on the shore of the pristine lake
30 feet away, talking.
How could I not know he was in danger?
I always did when he was young
and in his crib at night.
I'd stir from the slightest sound that was different
and lay awake or walk to his room
to make sure he was alive and still mine.
That day I heard the yelling. Maybe
even his cry sounding no different
from the normal commotion of the shoreline's children.
Jumping like Alice, he disappeared through the blue mirrored
water, and hit the rock that no one feared
then lost his way from life.
Drowning 30 feet away from where I sat talking.
I should have known my son was in danger because
I could have saved him.
Like I always did from his nighttime fears.
Now, I dream of his tearful calling.
Perplexed why I sit, unmoving and stare.

# *Observations, Insights, & Remembrances*

# Why?

## Why him, her, them?

If only there was a simple key that could be turned to make sense of this death and bring immediate healing... There is a simple key, but there isn't instant healing. The key to dealing with why your loved one died is acknowledging his death has occurred—whether it is from illness, an accident, old age, or violence. The person whom you lived with, loved, hated, cared for—is now gone. The outcome is always the same. Your life is forever changed. Adjusting to this change takes time and effort. There is no instant fix; no one page to read for answers.

Because there isn't instant healing, immediate acceptance of his death may not be possible. A more realistic goal is learning to accommodate to the changes in your life the death of your loved one brings, and finding ways to live with these sudden differences.

Life-altering changes require time for adjustment. Unfortunately, their impact on your everyday life will not wait until you're ready, but instead will feel like a dam that began leaking as soon as his death occurred. As water escapes through a dam, your daily life capabilities appear to be draining, often missing.

**Before the death, you probably weren't used to doing things like:**

—Forgetting your keys.

—Walking into a room on an errand only to find yourself standing aimlessly, forgetting what you came to do.

—Missing the turn into your driveway.
—Forgetting to bathe or eat.

It's tempting to criticize yourself – *I shouldn't be forgetting my keys!* – the hope being that if you were doing something wrong, this criticism will force you to simply change and do it right.

But loss is not fixed by a simple change in your actions. Loss burrows deep into your being. If you understand this, your inability to do things like remembering even automatic, simple tasks, can be understood. Your actions can be seen as a direct result of your mind, body and spirit trying to adjust to loss. You can stop being afraid. This is where accommodation can provide you with a bridge over your confusion.

Accommodation begins with becoming aware of what's *not* working; and as a result, making you aware of your changed needs and presenting you with solutions for dealing with them.

—Your memory will be overtaxed following a death. If you can't remember (even if memory is usually one of your strong points) make a list of everyday things.

—If you have not driven or are not in the right frame of mind to drive, ask for help getting rides.

—The need for sleep is paramount in healing. If you're unable to get enough sleep on your own; under a doctor's guidance, you might try medication to relax or to help you sleep.

—If your loved one was your partner and you struggle with sleeping alone, you might sleep with her pajamas next to you.

—If you are not bathing, eating, or getting dressed, you might leave yourself reminder notes until your concentration and motivation return.

—While you are getting used to her absence, you might need to carry on conversations with your loved one—be they angry conversations or ones in which you ask for guidance. It's okay.

—As you are learning to negotiate your way in the world without her, you might want the companionship of a pet.

—As you adjust, be open to adjusting your normal routines. You might cook less, clean less, simplify your commitments, take naps, find a hobby exercise. Guide your adjustments with compassion for yourself.

There are many ways to accommodate to the innumerable situations in which you'll find your life has changed. Pay attention to yourself. By paying attention, the seemingly alien landscape of your new everyday world will gain familiarity, and with that familiarity will come the ability to accept what has changed in your life. It won't happen all at once. It will happen in pieces as you process, then live with, then process again...

## HE KISSED HER

Alice died by the moonlight.
Quiet
after months of pain.
Her husband sat by her side,
holding her hand,
remembering their first touch,
how alive and free
he felt.
The moon's cool light
illuminating all that had been in shadow.
The months of his own pain
took shape, took hold.
He looked at her face.
His new found aloneness
perfectly reflected, stared back.
He wept.

*Observations, Insights, & Remembrances*

# Borrowing the Future

## If I knew then what I know now, I would have...

As humans, we look at events based on our life experience. It's tempting to believe that we should have known all along what we learned from the dying experience.

**The truth is, what you know now, you didn't know then:**

—How could you have known the cough wasn't a cold, but cancer?
—How could you have known something bad was going to happen when he went out in the car for the one-thousandth time?
—How could you have known a violent killer waited for her in the parking garage one mile from your home?
—How could you have known morphine would reduce her suffering in those last weeks, and that you didn't need to fear she would become addicted?

Hindsight is seductive. It holds the allure of failed omniscience. A bad, tragic, and sorrowful thing has happened to someone you love. There is no way you could have known it was going to happen. Your pain isn't necessarily a sign you did something wrong or that you failed. It is an affirmation that you have feelings and continue to love, that death doesn't erase your affection.

## GRANDSON

Grandson, dear,
your dark eyes show desperation,
as if our relationship
needs your efforts to keep me breathing and peaceful.
As if an extra minute would define our love—
it doesn't. I'll die happy.
Culling the knowledge of eighty years
into my 30-second flight
collapsing into God.
Wrap your arms around your marriage,
search for your children
whose smiles you seldom see.
Go home, grandson, go home.
Your family needs a grownup man.
I need the quiet to die.

## *Observations, Insights, & Remembrances*

## Complicated Grief

### A simple death can turn into a complicated parting when unfinished business from life remains.

Unfinished business from a relationship is like a splinter in the skin of your emotional life. Some issues pierce painfully deep, while others are barely under your emotional skin. Throughout your life, but especially at the end, your emotional splinters need to be located and pulled.

One place to look for them is in your important relationships. Deep emotional splinters can be found in relationships that are disrespectful. The disrespect might have occurred during childhood, or from an abusive relationship during adulthood. And the forms of disrespect can vary– it can be verbal, emotional, physical, sexual, or stem from neglect.

Relationships that are disrespectful can leave you feeling empty or numb, or opposite that, can sometimes leave you with intense feelings. If you feel either or both of these emotional extremes when examining a particular relationship, it tells you that something about the relationship needs tending to. It's very probable that you're dealing with a relationship that was at the least disrespectful. It might have been an abusive relationship.

In your examination of your important relationships, unfinished business can also be found in relationships that are solid and healthy. Moments of regret are few. Often, the unfinished business comes from things you wish you had said or done differently. These relationships have emotional splinters that barely pierce the skin. Their issues can be dealt with by simple gesture, word or deed.

If you are dying and have unfinished business, begin examining your significant relationships. Then decide which relationships and what kinds of issues you want to resolve. In your self-examination, ask yourself as honestly as you can, "How healthy, or wounded, am I feeling in each of my relationships?"

Use your thoughts and feelings about the relationship as your guide for answering this question. After acknowledging the issues and deciding which of your relationships you need to deal with, begin communicating. You can talk, text, write, or use any other form of communication that allows you to connect with each person in a way that is respectful of your and his or her needs. If the issues are painful and too scary to address with the person on your own, consider involving someone you trust to be there with you, like a counselor or a close friend. Since communicating directly may be a new experience, you may feel awkward or emotional. This is normal.

If you are experiencing the death of someone you love, your relationship may no longer be worked out person to person. This doesn't mean you are stuck with your feelings. It means you accept what you feel and think as an intimate part of who you are. These thoughts and feelings are messages from inside of you, trying to make their way out to be heard by you. They contain much needed information and learning from them strengthens you, allowing you to accept your present needs as important. Listening honestly to what you feel and think is a necessary kindness you will need to show yourself. It will help you to understand how to face the unique changes death has brought to your future. Strength doesn't come without struggle and pain.

When you are unable to work things out face to face, you can promote your healing by writing, thinking, reading, and talking with others who will listen. An example of this is writing to your loved one. Even if your loved one has already died, the letter can still be an effective way to communicate. It helps you to organize the unfinished business you have in your conscious mind. It allows you to say the things you still need to say.

Allow your letter to be heard. You might read it to his headstone.

Tie it to a balloon and let it be carried to the sky. Read it to someone you love. Talk about the feelings the letter made you aware of. Consistently reach out to those who care.

Sometimes the only way to resolve your unfinished business is to search out a good counselor. This is true when unfinished business has been harbored for a long time, and especially true when it is painful. Use these discussions with them as a compass to move your search for healing toward the actions you need to take to integrate your loss into personal strength, awareness, and health.

## AWKWARD TIMES ON EARTH

Your vengeance,
how can it stay living?
How can the stories remain fresh of all who failed you?
The bigotry speak with the verbal ease of a drunken tongue
that rudely tells the stories of the bald hairdresser with red
suspenders and
the homeless man with his curbside sexual tauntings.
How can you move in this darkness and
not desire to linger at the window in awe of the sunset?
Not pull your daughter closer,
making whole your fractured love.
How can you not ask forgiveness from the spirit of this world
for your part in concealing its mystery?
How will you move to the moment
when all your movement stops forevermore?
That moment is close, barely tucked in the future,
will it be just another awkward meeting?

# *Observations, Insights, & Remembrances*

# Finding Yourself

## What do I do with myself, now that I am without you?

It is not unusual, when you have intimately cared for someone who is dying, to think of your caretaker roles first, and your personal needs second. Your caretaker roles may have evolved into your temporary identity.

**Following your loved one's death, you'll experience moments like these:**

—I was on my way home when it hit me; I didn't have to be home at a certain time.

—I was near the pharmacy when I realized I didn't have to live around her medication schedule anymore.

—I was at the grocery store when it came to me that I didn't have to buy her special foods.

—Driving to my doctor's appointment, I realized I won't be her transportation to the doctor anymore.

These times of awareness are moments of clarity, where you can see that your life is forever and fundamentally different. Who are you without the roles? Facing this tough question may bring about intense emotions. To answer this, you first need to know that, though your life has permanently changed, your needs and personal dreams still exist.

**Begin to rediscover your individual needs and dreams by re-examining your earliest moments of clarity:**

—What thoughts and feelings occurred after you realized you were released from your caretaker role?

—Even if you felt guilty thinking it, were there things you looked forward to doing?

—Were there activities and people you knew you would miss?

—How full did your life seem?

In the process of focusing on your thoughts and answering the questions they raise, you will be able to reflect back on your original needs and aspirations. What have you done in the past to meet your needs and life's purpose? Were you able to meet them in healthy ways? If you weren't, do you need help to learn how?

Rediscovering and focusing on your life after a major loss can be a mixture of emptiness and freedom; two feelings that may seem incompatible, like water and oil.

If you feel free and are trying to uncover your future, does that mean you are being disrespectful and forgetting your shared past? ***No.*** Does it mean you are glad she has died? ***No.***

This has been a hard time. You are still alive. Your lifelong dreams are your path into the future.

## FOLLOW ME

Follow me
across the threshold
with trepidation for the unfolding.
Follow me
hold love tight
with your open hand not moving.
Follow me
to find the stones
where the Styx first bubbles from the ground.
Follow me
from the shoes
of your daughter drying out life from dancing
through golden flowers that dreamed of blue and
sodden earth that warmed the sun's absence.
Follow me
in distant nights when
once again you will dream
in laughter that courts my memory with sheer joy.
Follow me
as I continue
in the soft blanket draped on a winter's night
in water finding thirst, in sleep quenching weariness
in pictures of glass that see through the eye.
Follow me
when your resistance rests
in all that is endless
knowing I still love
in the scent that stirs you
in the longing voice that answers.

# *Observations, Insights, & Remembrances*

## Holidays

### Holidays are supposed to be fun, right?

HOLIDAYS WILL NOW BRING a heightened awareness of loss. The Christmas tree lightings and ornaments, carolers, the menorah at Hanukkah, the Thanksgiving feast, fireworks on the Fourth of July, trick-or-treaters, and the haunting rhythm of "Auld Lang Syne" are all reminders. They are ever-present messengers of death and loss in never-ending lines and social traditions.

Your first holidays after the death will probably have stretches of intense sorrow. This is not an indicator that you are doing something wrong. Your sorrow is there because someone you love is gone.

It's healing to acknowledge your loss. Talk about him, cry, feel his presence while doing his traditional tasks. Reach out to friends and family.

Don't be afraid to modify your old traditions, just don't abandon them. Realize that doing things for the first time since his death will be a mixture of the familiar and the unknown, of deep sadness and joy.

When you are able, either this first holiday or the next, create something new within your old traditions. The "new" is a way to acknowledge and reintegrate your loved one into the festivities.

**Some ideas for doing this are:**

—Lighting a scented candle during dinner and remembering his scent and presence in your life.

—Offering a toast to him as you learn to live without him.

—Taking a walk in one of his favorite places during the holidays.
—Visiting his grave or sacred spot.
—Holding hands and saying a prayer.
—Setting a symbolic place for him at the dinner table.
—Looking at pictures from past holidays.

There is no right thing to do, or right way to do it. All that's important is doing things that hold meaning for you and your loved ones.

## THANKSGIVING DAY

I’ve done nothing wrong
although I’ve died.
The change from loving with widespread arms on this holiday
to living memories
as time enters years
and your heart stays burdened
with the task of living on . . .
I’m sorry.

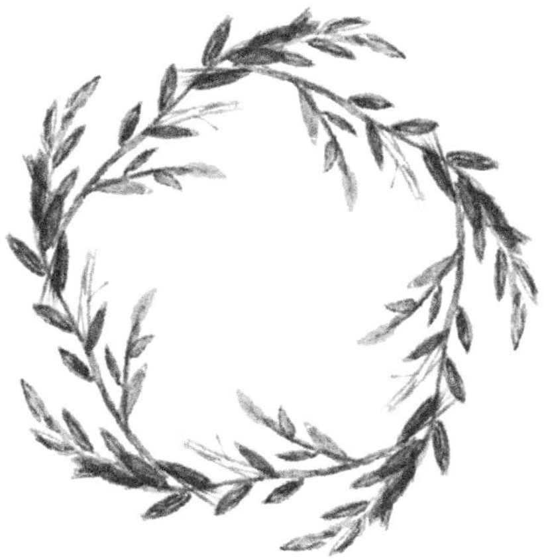

*Observations, Insights, & Remembrances*

## Adjusting to Your Changed Life

### Bereavement is not something that happens to you; but rather an experience that unfolds within you. The moments that will be especially difficult are called "firsts."

"FIRSTS" HAPPEN ANYTIME THAT you do something for the first time without your loved one, and they can trigger grief reactions.

Holidays are one kind of "firsts" that are easy to identify, anticipate and remember. Others, though, are more common and numerous than holidays. These "firsts" are difficult to anticipate, sometimes hard to identify, and especially powerful during the first year following a death.

Begin to compile your own list of "firsts." This record will help you anticipate what might trigger your grief feelings and enable you to feel a little less surprised and battered when they occur.

**Start your list by remembering what reminds you of being together, then group it into categories; such as:**

—Music and songs that have memories for you are especially potent—the first time you hear one that reminds you of her can bring a flood of emotions.

—Places you associate with your loved one—the first time you go there will bring back fond and emotional memories.

—People who knew both of you—when you carry on these relationships, the first time can bring strong feelings of loss, loneliness, and change.

—Foods that he loved—when you prepare them, eat or see them the first time, it's like tasting the emotions of your loss.

—Junk mail that is still addressed to him will keep arriving—the first time this happens will make clear that even the mundane of everyday life has been changed by his death; and can result in some overwhelming sadness.

Connecting your feelings to your "firsts" can help you make better sense of these emotional moments. The "firsts" can seem endless, but they're not. They won't go on forever.

## REMEMBERING

In the first months,
I waited with dinner.
I saw you in your autumn colored sweater
ten paces ahead, just out of reach,
never turning to my call;
disappearing
when I remembered.
In the first months,
I wrapped my pillow
with your bedclothes.
I smelled your skin and dreamed of your touch,
a lazy arm around my side as we slept.
Your breasts comfortable, nestled in the hollow of my back.
I knew you were there, until I remembered.
In the first months,
the days were torn open each time
I walked in the rhododendron park.
I lingered in the vegetable aisle.
I drove by the restaurant that furnished take out.
Each time, the first time, I was forced to live without you,
I remembered,
I remembered . . .

# *Observations, Insights, & Remembrances*

# Chapter Three

## Self-care and Meditation

TAKING CARE OF YOURSELF is one of the most challenging necessities during the times of great stress that go with bereavement. This chapter will give you some suggestions and exercises to aid in your self-care. Recognizing that it's not always possible to have an ideal time, many of these exercises can be used while you're active. You need only learn them to apply them in a variety of circumstances.

It is crucial that you take time to exercise, rest and reflect—finding rest and relief in the middle of heartache is a fundamental need. The greatest care you can give to others can only happen when you take great care of yourself.

**This chapter will teach you:**

—How to be aware of and understand your feelings.
—How to find your focus, even within chaos.
—How to reduce and manage stress.

## Surprising Emotions

Your feelings are neither right nor wrong, they are just your inner conversation. This conversation can guide you even when it might surprise you.

Feelings can be a mystery, a source of strength, a truth or a scary annoyance. To understand your feelings, know they are like a barometer for your inner world. They are neither right nor wrong, but simply information. It's like being thirsty. You wouldn't judge your thirst as being right or wrong but rather as an expression of need for the state of your body. Feelings are an expression of your psychological body.

During the events that take place when someone is dying, there is the desire to keep your feelings peaceful, or at least manageable, but the opposite typically happens. During intense times, your feelings will be more extreme. This can be scary when what you think you should feel carries little weight with what you do feel. If you become afraid, try not to run from or silently contain your stronger feelings because you will be denying yourself important information that will help you define your needs. Tending to your needs is the only way to ease your stress, which in turn, will make you better able to cope with the events taking place in your life.

## SEA OF FEELINGS

It was a morning first
hardened by sadness.
Its invisible walls, protecting,
me, an exhausted swimmer
from being swallowed by the wind-swept sea.
Although the possibility could be
it was me who had become the hurricane!
Learning you died, my love once tender
wanted only to wail!
So walls went up protecting the city,
the wind-swept sea, its level surging,
would bring devastation to no one
but those who loved you.
Those who loved you included me!

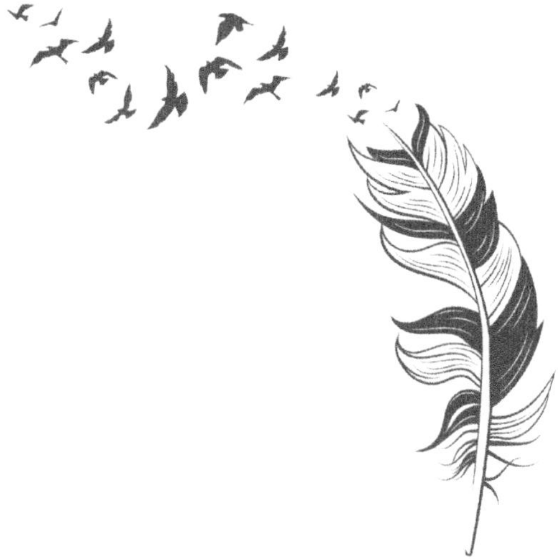

*Observations, Insights, & Remembrances*

## Indications That You're Feeling

### Since feelings tell you how you are and what you need, how do you know you're feeling?

**There are numerous signs, both emotional and physical, that will tell you when you are feeling:**

—General moodiness.
—Numbness.
—Snapping at people.
—Overdoing and/or underdoing—different from your normal behaviors when you are not under this kind of stress (e.g., overdrinking, over/under eating, over/under sexual activity, over/under sleeping).
—Physical signs, such as a racing heart, feeling sweaty, difficulty concentrating, memory lapses, or an upset stomach.
—Statements like; *I shouldn't be feeling*... If you are doing this, accept that *you are feeling* what you think you shouldn't be. It's you and it's true. Remember, it's simply information.

To determine what you might be feeling, try hard not to judge yourself. It doesn't do any good.

Once you realize that you *are* feeling, then hopefully you'll discover what those feelings are specifically; for it's important to develop ways to cope with your feelings and their effects on you.

## CARING

Behind his eyes
another moment spills open
in the mosaic piles of sorrow and knowing
its whisper must be seductive how else
could a 3 year old agree to die if
the earth were spiritless and the ground
only silent.
Its whisper
cooled his fever with explanations that mattered
so he relaxed without falling. His mother's arms
found his shape
and cooed memories so his heart
could finally rest after struggling, and struggling
and fading.
He was bathed in lavender soap,
there would be no more night sweating. He peacefully
folded into his best blue jeans and sweater
carried by his family on the parting walk
that keeps the spirit whole and present
in the memories we share.
He was soft, life was still hopeful
even in this beginning of whispers first heard without believing
they'd be left alone.

# *Observations, Insights, & Remembrances*

## Intense Feelings Aren't Necessarily Bad Feelings

### What I feel is so different from what I normally feel; I fear what will happen if I allow myself to hear them.

Remember that feelings are statements about our internal selves. Powerful feelings occur during times of life-changing events. Listening to what you feel will make you healthier in the long-run.

**Even though these strong feelings can seem frightening, there are ways to lessen their intensity:**

—Exercise.
—Keep a journal.
—Talk to others so feelings don't bottle up.
—Accept your feelings as important information.
—Talk with a counselor or support group if they get to be too much to understand or handle.

**Sometimes, intense feelings will lead to a physical need for expression; when your emotions are too difficult to contain, do something physical:**

—Exercise.
—Chop wood.
—Bang a stick against a tree.
—Hit a tennis racket on the bed.
—Smash a pillow with your fist.

Find whatever physical outlet is acceptable and comfortable for you. *(The rule always for the physical expression of your feelings is—do not hurt yourself or someone else.)*

Your feelings are an inward expression of a difficult and fundamental change in your life. Be kind to yourself and listen to them for direction.

## A WEEK AGO YOU WERE WELL

Fifty-three years of life,
of my life, has been a cushion.
I've not wanted you to fall
from the living,
from our loving and living together.
Living our lives with the convertible top down.
Feeding on the orange of an early morning sun,
shooting forward on some desert road.
On desert time we've lived.
Our together is rich, our together has defined us,
our has been my eyesight so much I can't see me.
I can't see you either—
you're collapsing inward,
slipping inward to a place that knows neither of us.
I can't contain this thinking.
One thought ignites another!
If only I could scream
on a high, deserted rock.
Screaming at a new moon
to appear from its darkness.
Maybe I could find me?
Maybe I could hear my name and
bear your final touch. Before death's journey with you alone.
Yet, here we are
in the heat, two flights up with no fan working.
The convertible is parked.

## *Observations, Insights, & Remembrances*

## Ways Stress Can Impact Us

### Losing yourself in the stress of seeing your loved one die.

Living with the demands of a terminal illness can slowly change how you determine if you are okay. It can cause you to connect how you feel emotionally with how the terminal illness is doing physically. You might think the two are the same; they're not, but one can impact the other.

Physical pain is usually measurable—it's sharp or dull, severe or mild. It can come with other physical symptoms as well, like nausea, fever, elevated heart rate and rapid breathing. Emotional pain can come as a result of caring for someone with constant physical pain. It's experienced through sadness or depression, anxiety or anger, not feeling enough or too much.

When you are feeling, your emotions provide you with two types of information. One, how you are in the here and now. The other, how you've been as you have lived your life over time. Physical symptoms of a terminal illness strictly relate to the here and now. Living with the immediate and long-term demands of a physical illness stimulates intense feelings. Without conscious effort, this intensity will dull your sense of self. Living this way day in and day out can leave you forgetting who you are. Sadness can turn into depression and feelings of hopelessness. You can lose your desire to participate, your hope that you can manage, your sense of well-being. When you're emotionally overwhelmed, your usual ways of engaging in and enjoying life can seem like they require too much effort.

Remember, your emotional self is separate from the illness. To refocus on your emotional self, begin by defining two terms—*internal focus of control* and *external focus of control.*

**Internal focus of control:** Knowing how you are doing by looking inside yourself. It involves being aware of what you're feeling and thinking—which lets you know how you are.

—Sometimes when I feel afraid, I think of places that I love. Remembering them usually helps me to relax.

—I can feel myself getting tense, so I step outside for fresh air.

—It feels really good to cry.

—I remember something she told me last year. Thinking of it helps me as I sit alongside her bed.

**External focus of control:** Determining how you are doing by how people and events are acting or reacting around you. If people are okay, then you're alright; but if there's conflict outside of you, it creates conflict inside of you.

—I worry that my pain will upset everyone... so I keep it to myself.

—I feel like I'm walking on eggshells.

—I look around the living room to where his bed is. I have to make sure no one is crying and upsetting him.

—The heat in the room is too high. My relatives are too loud. I want to go home, but I have to make sure everyone in the room is okay.

If it's difficult to identify what your focus is, conduct a survey. At different times of the day, take a minute to see how you are doing by reviewing recent events in the day. Were you mostly tending to other's feelings and needs, therefore unaware of your own? This is externally focused. Staying externally focused keeps you distracted and away from yourself, and tied to the physical illness. It is a powerful way to keep you on edge and highly stressed.

Were you able to listen to your needs? Did you take some time away from care giving to do something for yourself? This is being internally focused, and allows you to separate your emotional self from the physical illness. Even under stress, it will help you know what you need to do to take care of yourself and maintain your emotional health.

## DOUBLE TO SINGLE BED

Holding your back, arranging the pillows.
Kissing the memories from
your mouth and cheeks and decades
of health now twisted behind and hidden
in this month of endless waking
in an electric bed with hospital sides
that keep you from harm
and me forever reaching through its cold metal bars.
Reaching past your dying and into those memories
that barely fill my emptiness
for what we used to be.

*Observations, Insights, & Remembrances*

## Listening Inside

### An internal focus for control can be developed.

SIT OR STAND QUIETLY. Be aware of the outline of your body. The outline of your body is where you physically begin and the world outside ends. It is where the internal focus of control begins and the external ends.

When under stress, the outline of your body can become like a wall that keeps events and others at a distance. Tension comes from maintaining your wall. It takes emotional energy to both call it into place and to keep it there. Expending emotional energy for survival tasks brings on tension. If the outline of your body feels like a wall, mentally experiment with giving it gates or windows. Give yourself permission to open them. Visualize opening them. Think of light and fresh air coming in. Feel them restoring and relaxing you.

At first, you might do this exercise for short periods of time. Gradually increase the time you do it. Once you've practiced this exercise a couple of dozen times sitting quietly, practice it in the middle of your activities. Using this mental exercise of opening your inner windows redeems your emotional energy for other uses, such as relaxing. Relaxing in the midst of difficult times in life will make you better able to cope with the stress and difficult tasks you have to deal with.

Opening your windows helps you to restore a productive sense of balance. It is your choice and effort to control how and when they will open.

## SHIRTLESS

I listen,
the sun penetrates
and warms my skin.
I call to you, Father
my shoulders hunched
placing a boundary for
the tired numbness
that fills me
like a low morning fog.
With the forgotten
understanding that you speak
not bound by words
but in the sun
and on the wind.
I listen, shirtless.

*Observations, Insights, & Remembrances*

# Relaxation Exercises

## In times of active stress, relaxation must be active, too.

THE GOAL OF THIS exercise is to physically drain stress away. It can be done anywhere, whether sitting, standing, or lying down—don't worry, others won't know what you're doing. This exercise, known as progressive muscle relaxation, involves the tension and relaxation of each body part; finishing with the whole body being tensed, then relaxed.

### Progressive Muscle Relaxation

—Starting with your face, head, and neck, gradually tense them. Clench your jaw. Scrunch your eyes closed. Tense your cheeks. Hold this tension for 10 to 15 seconds. Burn up the stress. Then relax them. Let your jaw drop and your face sag. Focus on and learn the difference between tension and relaxation in this part of your body.

—Go to your neck, shoulders, arms, hands, and chest. Tighten them by clenching your fists, flexing the muscles of your chest and arms, and scrunching up your neck. Hold this position for 10 to 15 seconds. Burn up the stress. Then relax them. Focus on and learn the difference between tension and relaxation in this part of your body.

—Go to your stomach. The stomach, chest and jaw are often where the noticeable effects of stress reside. Tighten the muscles of your stomach—making them into steel. Hold this position for 10 to 15 seconds. Burn up the stress. Then relax your stomach and let it soften. Focus on and learn the difference between tension and relaxation in this part of your body.

—Go to your legs and feet. Tense them. Make your feet into tight balls. Make your legs into tree trunks. Hold this position for 10 to 15 seconds. Burn up the stress. Then relax your legs and feet. Focus on and learn the difference between tension and relaxation in this part of your body.

—Tense every part of your body—your face, neck, chest, stomach, buttocks, legs, and feet. Feel the tension in your entire body. Hold this position for 15 to 20 seconds. Burn up the stress. Then relax. Feel what it is like to consciously relax every part of your body.

This exercise should allow you to feel more physically and mentally relaxed. You now possess awareness and a tool. The awareness comes from how your body feels when it's tense while under stress, and it's a cornerstone to gaining an internal focus of control. Part of the internal focus comes from knowing how and what your body is doing. When your body tension tells you that you are under stress, that's the time to check in with yourself to see what's causing it. Knowing what's causing it will help you develop a plan for dealing with it.

When you're really overwhelmed or don't see yourself as having the luxury of developing a plan, you still need to take care of yourself. This exercise can help you in that essential care.

# MEDITATION

Simple
breath
mild
exhortations
with
no effort
old dynasties
fall.

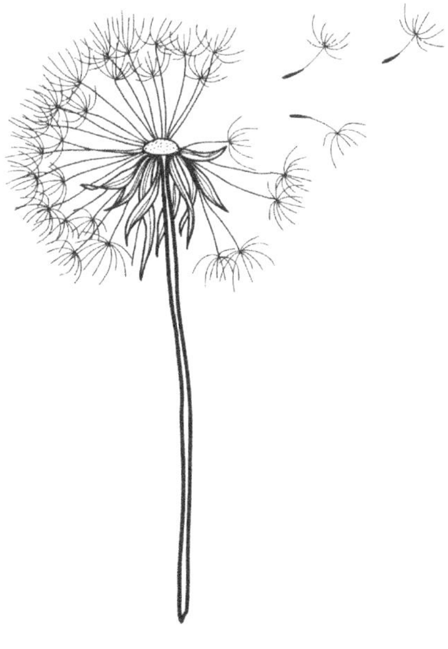

## *Observations, Insights, & Remembrances*

# Not a Well-paved Road

## On your road to a rediscovered life, there will be potholes.

THE DAY WILL COME when you will feel like you have hit a rut, lost control and driven off the road. The experience can be overwhelming enough to make you think you are back to the first days of grieving.

Events that trigger grief are easily overlooked. Hard days often revolve around overlooked "firsts." When you feel strongly and it isn't clear why, you've probably not been aware of a "first" within your day.

**Look for and reflect on some possible reasons for your overwhelming feelings:**

—Examine the calendar.
—Search the calendar of memories in your heart.
—Reflect upon what you've been doing, where you've been, or where you are anticipating going.
—Think about the people you've been in contact with, or will be in the presence with soon.

Are any of these days, situations, memories, or people connected to your loved one?

**By reflecting, it is not unusual to suddenly remember that:**

—You heard her special song.
—You saw a glimpse of your mother's face in an actress while watching a movie.
—Over the weekend, you cleaned his area of the closet for the first time.
—This morning, you found his pocket knife.
—You stumbled upon and read his old love letters.

When you know what has triggered your feelings, you can deal with them. Knowing how to recognize and accept the information your feelings bring are solid skills for making it through new situations. When you make the connection between what you are feeling and what triggered your feelings, you will experience the difference between early stage and late stage grief. Early grief has no boundaries and no ability to understand anything but pain. Late stage grief diminishes when you recognize its trigger and do what is needed to take care of you.

Rediscovering how to make your life work is an ongoing effort of reflection and processing. The effort pays off, though, as living becomes easier, your outlook more optimistic. When difficult days inevitably still arise, be confident that you haven't fallen backwards—you're only having a tough day. Most days are better, but today is not.

## ALWAYS THERE

On a glass track
steaming toward an absent moon
a lone train whistle cries out for humanity.
From the bottom land
of unredeemed losses,
from the junctures plowed
with then and now and random songs
that whistle through life's marrow.
I heard its call
when you spoke
of his brushing touch
soft with love
and emptied life,
save the memories
that pulse in your heart
like comfortable ghosts
not restrained by rules, or form, or shadows.

*Observations, Insights, & Remembrances*

## Parenting After Loss

### I'm no longer just surviving. What can I now do to understand my child and aid her with her healing.

REMEMBER THAT CHILDREN ARE little people—as capable of experiencing the similar depths of emotion as grown ups. Being little, they simply don't always have the verbal communication skills to discuss what is on their minds and in their hearts.

Even though their verbal skills may not be developed, their ability to feel is. They experience the same pain, emptiness, and other feelings spawned by death.

When children don't have the skills to verbally communicate their feelings, they'll show them to you. You can make a guess about their feelings by reflecting on their actions. Is anything out of the ordinary? Is there an escalation of the ordinary? Are they withdrawn or acting out? View changes from the norm as a statement of feelings.

There are things you can do to help them to express their feelings and communicate their needs. Do not hesitate to use community resources or get a professional opinion if you need guidance. This could be at a grief center with a support group, or a professional who specializes in working with bereavement and children.

Create opportunities for you and your child to interact specifically around the death. You both can make a "memory box," where he can place select objects that remind him of the person who died. Don't screen what goes in the box. Encourage him to talk about the items and their connection to the one who died. By talking about his loss, he will be expressing himself and giving form to his feelings.

After all the objects are selected, provide him with materials to decorate the inside and outside of the box. As he is doing it, have him tell you what the decorations mean to him. This box will now serve as a place for him to go to when he needs to be close and remember. It gives him a place to focus on his feelings, while giving both of you a safe and predictable way to come together around the loss. Part of remembering is having fragments of the lost relationship become tangible and present again.

You might consider making your own memory box and sharing your memory items with your child. It validates his feelings to hear you express your own. Keep your expression in line with his age and developmental level. He can be helped in his own understanding of his loss when he hears you work on yours. Be careful and remember your child isn't your counselor.

Find books on your child's level that deal with death. Read them together and talk about whatever comes up. Art projects can help bring feelings to the surface. Draw pictures together of your loved one, or the places you visited with them. You could also cut pictures from a magazine and make a collage.

## BOX

I'd been afraid to unwrap the tinfoil
I tightened almost two years ago
around the rock I'd lifted
from your grave.
Stopping from shoveling
the dark wet clay,
I picked up this opulent white rock
that glistened in the rain.
In it, I heard you whisper.
In this box of memories,
decorated with a mummified red rose and
a paper plate that carried the last meal we shared,
has been your rock, unopened and waiting;
until today.
To untangle the memory of your warmth
I'll unwrap the rock and free
your whispering from that day, a conversation that's not ended.
Whisper again, I know you will.
Free in spirit,
alive in my box of memories.
I'll open it when I need to feel your living presence.
Whispering is okay
for the language of remembering.
Whispering is okay. I'm not afraid to listen today.

# *Observations, Insights & Remembrances*

## New Relationships

Starting a new relationship can be scary.

It is important to remember you are still alive. It's easy to forget what this really means immediately following the death of your loved one. Your daily needs were simplified; as you need only to cry, think, sleep, talk and eat.

Just as an eclipse of the sun doesn't last forever, sorrow eclipsing the fundamental needs of life won't either. Eventually, their light will be seen. You can ignore them or attempt to make yourself feel guilty for having them, but neither of these solutions are healthy, nor will they be effective for long.

It is more helpful to learn about and acknowledge what your needs are. You can do this by listening to your thoughts—even those in passing. Discover what you are drawn to. Often your needs are quite straightforward; consisting of expressing and receiving love, feeling valued, creating, and finding renewed purpose.

Many times these needs take shape in the desire to be in a relationship of some kind again. This happens because companionship is a fundamental need for most of us.

**Beginning a new relationship after your partner dies seems like a near-impossible task, filled with many questions and unknowns:**

—How do I meet someone?
—How do I date someone after not dating for thirty years?
—What kind of person am I attracted to?

—How do I decide if a person is okay to date?

—How do I shed the guilt I feel when I think of being with a different person?

The unknowns appear as dangerous and frightening as tightrope walking without knowing how. To gain confidence, begin cultivating an understanding of yourself as a single person. What are your likes and dislikes, hobbies and interests? What are your strengths and weaknesses?

The thought of dating might make you feel guilty—like you are betraying your loved one. It's important to remember that *you* are still living. Life continues to tug at your sleeve asking you not to withdraw for too long. Life still knows you, even though you have temporarily lost your understanding of its everyday possibilities and needs.

Many relationships that are established after a partner dies are based on companionship. Even though there may be frequent passion and the giddiness of new love, the bedrock of the relationship is compatibility.

If you think of your goal as compatibility, you understand that you need to find a friend. Establishing a compatible friendship is much less scary than the task of finding another true love and soulmate.

Guiding yourself toward compatible friendships is dependent on different factors. The main issues involve how inclusive or exclusive of others your relationship with your loved one was. If your relationship had included different individual friendships, finding compatible friendships will be easier. If your relationship minimized friendships with others, knowing how to be involved with others will be awkward and new.

Regardless of how inclusive or exclusive your relationship was, you now face the challenge of intimacy. For the first time in what might be a long time, you are free to begin a new committed relationship.

The expectations you have from your previous relationship might lead you to believe that most new relationships are capable of commitment and deep intimacy. But in reality, what worked in your previous relationship is not automatically transferable to a new relationship. Intimacy is a journey of trust, not an immediate destination, and not all friendships are capable of this kind of commitment.

A tool for evaluating your relationships is in the following diagram. Use this chart to help yourself weigh how and how often intimacy might develop.

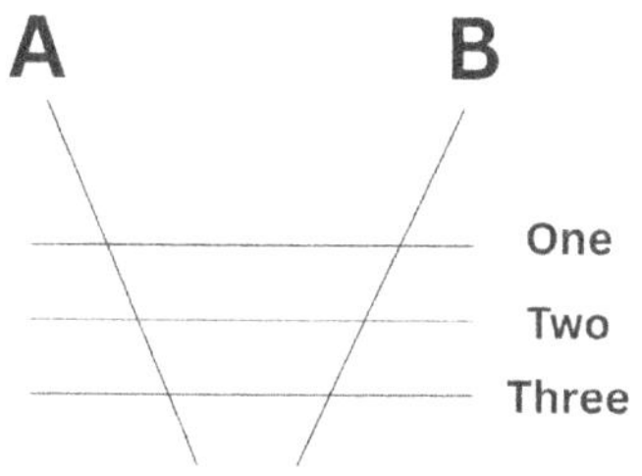


Lines one, two and three of the diagram represent levels of intimacy. Line one represents everyday relationships—people you say hello to, and talk about the weather. There is little revealed about your deeper thoughts, your fears or dreams. Trust is there, but it is guarded; thus, intimacy is minimal.

Line two has greater compatibility and trust than line one. There is some deeper sharing, but private thoughts and feelings are kept mostly to yourself.

A deeper level of trust distinguishes line three. On this relationship level, you can talk openly about your feelings, deeper thoughts and aspirations. You can risk looking vulnerable because it's balanced with the other's knowledge of your good qualities. Level one relationships have minimal or unexplored compatibility and intimacy. Level three relationships have great compatibility and deeper intimacy.

The down lines A and B are like the top of a funnel. They represent the number of people available to be involved in a relationship with you. At the top, by line one, is the greatest number of people. You can and will have many level one relationships. As follow the lines down to the bottom of the funnel, there are significantly fewer people who can be in a level three relationship with you.

Think about your relationships. What qualities of trust do they possess? Are they level one, two or three?

You may find yourself trying to make a level one or two relationship into a level three, but it can't be forced. Level three will only happen over time. So, if you are in a level one relationship and have been trying to meet your level three needs, you're probably going to become frustrated. New relationships begin at level one, rarely at level three.

Knowing how commitment and intimacy develops within relationships, you can now temper your expectations. If you want level three relationships, they can happen over time. Creating them involves taking risks and remaining open to your needs for intimacy.

## LOVE AGAIN

One spring afternoon
a meadowlark sang
feathered in yellow down
singing on barbed wire grass
washed gray.
Its blue sky song reaching
corridors of memories
curled through life
that lead to love, again.
With echoes of you
I stop to listen

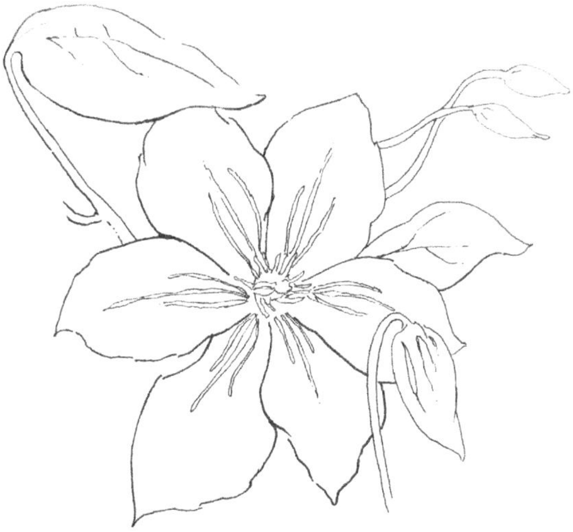

*Observations, Insights & Remembrances*

## Creating Meaning

The reminders of your loss can be used positively to create understanding.

REMEMBERING YOUR LOVED ONE is necessary and vital. During your private reflections, when the meaning of her death appears purposeless, inviting the community to remember with you can help. The goal is to find ways to honor your loss; thereby honoring your loved one, and helping others to benefit from your experience.

**There are numerous ways that might give meaning to your experience and honor your loved one's death:**

—Reread anything you wrote to her or about her—like your journal, blogs, texts or letters. Journals are a good way to see what you went through and how far you've come. Blogs are shared with others who might be able to benefit from your experience.

—Think back to what was going on during the dying process. Were there times when you needed help and it didn't exist? As you identify these times, you can think of ways that you might benefit others in similar situations. For example, a parent, whose daughter died of cancer, is able to identify situations during her illness when she could have used support. As a way of honoring her daughter and helping others, she formed a nonprofit organization to help other families, in the hospital and at home, in ways that her family needed help.

—Donate some of his books to the library. In the cover of the book, you can write an inscription; *In memory of...*

—Donate money to a favorite charity in her name.

—Host an event to raise money for a worthy cause. A family could host an annual bike ride to honor their daughter. The money is then donated to a charity in her name.

—Plant trees or a memorial garden in your loved one's name. Many families do this to benefit city parks, schools and even their own home.

Use your imagination and discover ways that allow your loved one's memory to live on. There is great solace to be found in simple acts of remembering.

## IN MEMORY

In memory of you,
I'd balance the moon
on the edge of a box.
But since I can't,
please know this flower that grows
was planted for you.
In memory of you,
I'd soar unassisted
showing even without wings
with love one can fly.
But since I'm unable,
know the ham radio you cherished
was put to use in the school.
In memory of you
I'd find a passageway to open
through the center of the earth.
But since that's not likely,
know that a family that suffered
receives help once a month.
In memory of you,
I'd create everything that could be
but my hands are only two.
So I'll find what might be small things
to make life better in some way.
In the process of doing them,
I will be remembering you.

## *Observations, Insights & Remembrances*

## Nature

When listening to nature, there are perspectives for healing and lessons leading to solutions for relearning how to live a changed life.

NATURE CAN GIVE YOU solace in your ongoing adjustment to the absence death creates. Its solitude gives time for reflection, remembering and thinking. In nature, you can observe the seasons of life, being reminded that even with the painful loss you've gone through, the seasons of life go on.

Go out, walk, sit, photograph, draw, paint, sing, be silent. In your silence, the wordless language of nature will help translate your grief into the everyday words of living.

## Loss is Everywhere

### At first, I could only remember her death.

WHEN YOU FIRST EXPERIENCE the death of someone you love, barely a minute goes by without thinking of it and your loss. The transition from having someone there physically to having them on the increasingly fragile threads of memory, is painful.

The constant thoughts about death painfully grind the gears of living—it seems that life will be like this forever. Life however, is forever changing. Life—because you are still living—goes on.

**In time, there will signs that begin to show that you're integrating your loss:**

—Realizing that you did not think of him for at least an hour.
—Finding yourself laughing again.
—Discovering renewed energy to accomplish daily tasks.
—Being more aware of others and their needs.
—Renewing old friendships and seeking opportunities for new ones.
—Feeling surprised at anticipating the future.

Eventually, and most importantly, healing is the move from remembering only his death to remembering mostly his life.

## SEASONS COME AND GO

It's warm
again. Snow appears like morning sleep
resting
on the mountains.
Shirtsleeve breezes
blow the scent of sap as it stretches
within the conifers.
Last year your absence
lay frozen
inside me. Its icy numbness
linked my days in toneless grays.
Winter seemed forever,
summer never came.
That's what makes today noticeable.
I feel life stirring!
My senses are penetrated by color.
You're not forgotten. Your loss
is still defining—it's that
your living is remembered. It stretches
within me.
Your scent
gathers with the breeze.

*Observations, Insights, & Remembrances*

## Generations

An integration of the generations appears in the vacuum created by death.

YOUR GRANDSON'S NOSE IS just like your husband's. One afternoon while looking in the mirror, you discover that your eyes are not only the same color as his, but have the same lashes, the same wrinkles and the same depth. Your daughter's smile and laugh reanimate your mom's. Your memories pop back to the times you remember your mother laughing.

Physical features are the most visible passage from death to life. They link your loved one to your family—they carry him through you into the present and future.

In time, his mannerisms will also surface. His sayings tumble out of your mouth at the moments that, if he'd been there, they might have come out of his. Some of the things he liked become the things you like even more.

Life is not only the shell of our body. It is the tangible and intangible substance that shows who we are and who we strive to be. His life, seemingly separate when he was alive, has crossed into the living generations by way of characteristics and character.

## DYLAN AND AVA

Salmon spawn
in the bedroom
surrounded by heavy wood
and the movement of the sea.
Two children emerge
from the water and soft skin with
the eyes of their deceased grandfather
reborn
after twenty years in the grave.

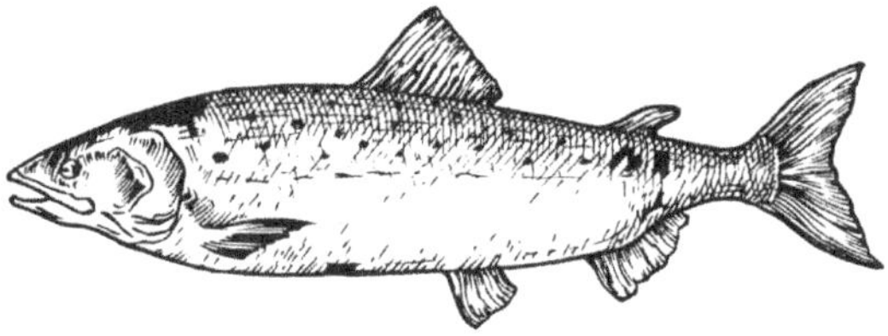

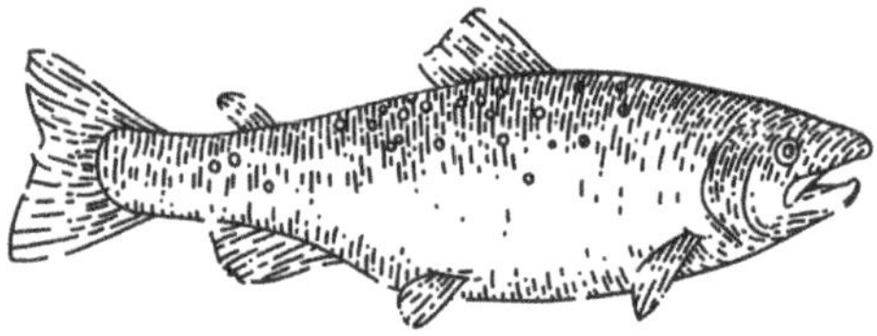

*Observations, Insights, & Remembrances*

## Struggle Creates a New You

### With all that you've been through, what do you own?

From your struggle, you've come to an understanding of yourself as you have accommodated to your loss. This understanding didn't happen to you, it happened through your efforts. Even though your efforts sometimes seemed like shining a flashlight at a distant star—wondering if its light would really make it there—the easing of your pain confirms that it did.

Because you own the understanding that has come through your efforts, you are a healthier person. Being healthy doesn't mean you don't feel or that you can control your feelings. It means that when you feel, you understand your feelings in context to what you are going through. Your emotions become a barometer for the internal and external events that are playing out in your life. Turning toward them is your strength.

The death of your loved one is a permanent change to your life. With the understanding you've gained, you realize joy can coexist with sorrow. From your hard work, the skills you've gained to understand and take care of yourself will always be available to you. The greatest of these skills is feeling whatever you are feeling. It is knowing that by feeling, you will have the clues for understanding your inner needs. By listening to and acting upon them, you can outgrow your pain.

## OUR BODIES CAST ASIDE

Maybe this life
is gestation.
Our bodies grow and become old
and lead us here like a newborn where
the Earth prepares for the arrival
of death with its silent cries.
In winter's blues
the Earth waits to spin
the horse haired knowledge of our lives.
To weave a blanket for sleep.
The efforts from birth
will deliver us weary.
Our efforts from loving
keep us always ready.

## *Observations, Insights, & Remembrances*

# Quiet

## In silence, take a few minutes to appreciate yourself.

In the stress you have been through, self-affirmations tend to get buried under the turmoil. Given the chance, you can probably recall five things that didn't go well. But it's essential to recognize and acknowledge what you *did do well.*

The most succinct way to recall the good things you did is in silence. You've been through a lot—the unimaginable is now part of your life experience.

When people go through difficult times, it is common for them to minimize what they have gone through. It's even easier to downplay the efforts made to get through it. Your efforts were meaningful and significant. What you have been through has been difficult and at times, nearly impossible. Despite it all, you made it. You have been wounded, but you survived. Your wounds—when tended to and acknowledged—are your future strengths.

A good way to develop an appreciation of you is to reflect in silence. Find a comfortable chair. Close your eyes. In your mind, say, *I appreciate my...* Fill in the blank with something you did, or handled, or naturally brought to the situation. With each remembrance, say again, *I appreciate my...* and complete the sentence with that remembrance of yourself and your efforts. Even if only one thing comes to mind, still do it. Then do it again on another day.

In healing from the turmoil, it is necessary to remember those qualities that make you a unique, caring, and loving person. Take a few minutes for silent affirmations.

## HOPE

When
there is no hope,
hope for inner sight
that can see
in the undistinguished acts that make up living,
meaning, and shows you to be,
in simplicity, whole.

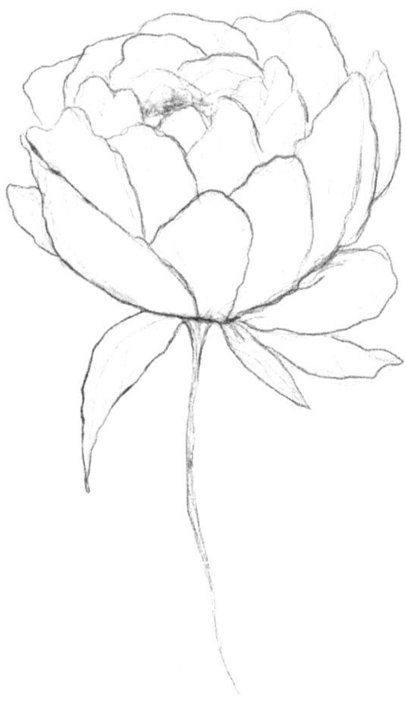

*Observations, Insights, & Remembrances*

# Living

## Your life will go on.

Now is the time for life to go on. How can it? It goes on by holding onto the memories from your past that are too crucial to let go. It can go on by assessing the present with open eyes. It will go on by dreaming, planning and living for the future.

**Here is a simple exercise:**

—Face in one direction. Stand or sit with your eyes closed. Think of this direction as facing the past. Remember those things from your past that are important—memories of times together, dreams and discussions, those qualities from your shared life that influence living today.

—Next, look at where you are, be aware of the spot where you are standing or sitting. This is the present. Experience your current strength and remembered sorrow. Listen to and feel your heartbeat. Your present is the engine, the vehicle you have for continuing in life. Raise your arms from your sides. Then fold them across your heart. You are pulling your past and present together.

—Now, turn and face the opposite direction. This is the future. You are not abandoning your loved one. You are not abandoning your shared dreams or the memories you created together. You are taking what you have identified as important, holding it close to your heart and bringing it with you. It is your source of strength, tenderness, empathy and direction. It is a part of you. You are your future.

What do you want your children, friends, loved ones, family and contemporaries to know and remember about you? Your life springs from you. One day others will hold inside what you have shown to be important in your living. One day, they too, will need to face the future—carrying you with them, living on.

## WHAT I WANT MY CHILDREN TO KNOW

The world is round,
the sky turns blue.
Roads are tarred.
The ground is deep.
Thinking guides you.
Feelings are food upon the table.
The heart does more than beat.
Mystery abides in eagle or wren.
God's presence radiates
from the bark of a tree.
The forgotten person has
life from which all living come.
Honor yourself and so honor others.
Love the pungent smell that makes you, you.
Find the love that's issued you.
Walk to the side of the tar that's on your path.
The ground is deep; the world stays round.
Mystery abounds in the heart that does more than beat.

*Observations, Insights, & Remembrances*

# Acknowledgements

This book would not be what it is without the talents of Ariane Kimlinger and Deanna DeLong. Their keen sense and sensitivities for the written word and for the reader, helped the quality of ***How to Live with Dying*** become more than what it would have been had it been left to me alone. I am grateful for their editorial skills and efforts—but mostly, for who they are as people.

**Artists:**

—Kay Harris (page 135)

—Maggie Hobson-Baker (pages 77; 81; 162; 174)

—Melanie Platt (page 12)

—Ava Sinead Zoebelein (page 58)

—Dylan Thomas Zoebelein (Chapters' Introduction woodblock)

—Maureen Zoebelein (Book cover; Observations... woodcut; page 141)

# About the Author

Tim Zoebelein, a clinical social worker for over thirty years, wrote this book out of a desire to help those who are facing the end of life. He spent twenty-three years at an Oregon hospice program in Portland, where he saw suffering and compassion; bravery while coping with overwhelming fear; and both abandonment and the coming together of family and friends. Tim's background includes the Peace Corps and public school teaching; and today, he maintains a private practice specializing in end-of-life and bereavement counseling.

Tim currently lives in Forest Grove, Oregon with his wife of fifty years. His two adult children live in Oregon as well. Always filled with the need to make the most of what he has as a human being, outside his practice, Tim enjoys meditation, hiking, getting together with friends, pottery, travel and woodworking.

The defining deaths in his life were the deaths of his father, who died when Tim was eighteen, his grandparents, his mother and friends.

"I consider myself overwhelmingly fortunate throughout my life; even when the sorrows I've gone through have temporarily laid me low."

JOY Rx

Children's Cancer Association

In memory of Alexandra Ellis, the
Children's Cancer Association (CCA)
was founded by her loving parents.

30% of the net proceeds from my book will
be donated to Children's Cancer Association

If you would like to make a donation
in support, please visit www.joyrx.org

Or mail it to:
Children's Cancer Association
1200 NW Naito Pkwy, Suite 140
Portland, OR 97209

Made in the USA
Coppell, TX
23 January 2026

69163869R00115